Read What Amazon Buyers Are S[a]
Certification Exam Q&A With Explanations books

- 5.0 out of 5 stars

By L. Mon March 2, 2016

Very easy to read and understand. Would definitely recommend to others.

- 5.0 out of 5 stars

By Crazy Mom on October 16, 2015

I highly recommend this for ACLS renewal review!!!! This is a great study guide for ACLS or renewal. I read all the practice questions the night before and received a 98% on the test. The analysis of each answer really helped me understand and retain everything. I have since shared it with co-workers when they are due to renew their ACLS.

- 5.0 out of 5 stars

By JetPowers on April 25, 2015

Focused toward passing the exam. Face it, even if we run codes these questions can be tricky – and try to keep up with the ever changing AHA guidelines. The pre-amble to test questions is well organized easy reading, useful and interesting. The test answers with explanations speak for themselves. It's a great pre-course study guide for passing the certification exam and focused for that purpose

- 5.0 out of 5 stars

By Mark on April 21, 2015

Easy to follow. An outstanding guide. Helped me pass the course, easy to follow!!!! Highly recommended!!

- 5.0 out of 5 stars

By VCRN on December 15, 2015

This is a comprehensive yet concise review book. I have to recertify every two years and found it a great refresher course of the details of practice that we are consistently tested on but may not stick in memory. I can also appreciate its value for the first time student. It gave me confidence to go into class confident I knew what I was doing and could convey that when tested. Highly recommend it!

Read What Amazon Buyers Are Saying About The
Certification Exam Q&A With Explanations books

• 5.0 out of 5 stars

By Karen McKinney on May 4, 2015

This book is excellent. There are many practice questions to get you prepared. Lots of practical and usable information and advice about the ACLS class and exam. I highly recommend this book. Get it! You and your patient will be glad you did.

• 5.0 out of 5 stars

By Mina Markazi on April 21, 2015

Excellent book.

• 5.0 out of 5 stars

By Dale C. Pickart on September 21, 2015

Very helpful!

• 5.0 out of 5 stars

By Amazon Customer on January 6, 2016

Would recommend for everyone taking ACLS. Excellent study guide.

• 5.0 out of 5 stars

By Jaws on November 20, 2015

Looks good. Bought to prep for exams.

• 5.0 out of 5 stars

By OneDiamondForever on February 16, 2016

Dead on!! A great review!!

• 5.0 out of 5 stars

By Donna Leonard on January 21, 2016

As advertised.

BLS
(Basic Life Support)

CERTIFICATION EXAM

Q&A

WITH EXPLANATIONS

FOR HEALTHCARE PROFESSIONALS AND STUDENTS
UPDATED USING THE LATEST GUIDELINES AND RESEARCH

Michele G. Kunz, MSN, ANP, RN-BC
& Joseph C. Kunz, Jr., MBA
Foreword by Dr. Thierry Duchatellier, MD

Dickson Keanaghan, LLC
Long Island, New York

Publisher: Dickson Keanaghan, LLC, Long Island, New York
Website: DicksonKeanaghan.com
Publication Date: April 01, 2017
Printed in the USA

College administrators and instructors, college bookstores, and book retailers, can order this book directly from Ingram.

Publisher's Cataloging-In-Publication Data

Names: Kunz, Michele G., author | Kunz, Joseph C. III., author. | Duchatellier, Thierry, foreword author.
Title: BLS (Basic life support) certification exam Q & A with explanations: for healthcare professionals and students, updated using the latest guidelines and research / Michele G. Kunz, MSN, ANP, RN-BC; Joseph C. Kunz, Jr., MBA ; foreword by Dr. Thierry Duchatellier.
Description: Includes bibliographical references. | Long Island, NY: Dickson Keanaghan, LLC, 2017.
Identifiers: ISBN 978-1-933230-80-1 | LCCN 2016919307
Subjects: LCSH Emergency medicine. | Life support systems (Critical care) | Medical emergencies. | First aid in illness and injury. | Emergency Medical Technicians--Education--Examination Questions. | Emergency Treatment--Methods--Examination Questions. | BISAC MEDICAL / Emergency Medicine | MEDICAL / Education & Training | MEDICAL / Test Preparation & Review
Classification: LCC RC86.7 .K86 2017| DDC 616.02/5--dc23

Table Of Contents

Note: Dickson Keanaghan developed this book to be a living, evolving document, and as such, intends to update this document as needed, and as new content becomes available. We welcome your participation to keep this book up to date. If you know of more recent developments, or have suggestions for other topics to cover within this publication, please let us know. Contact JCKunzJr@DicksonKeanghan.com.

Foreword

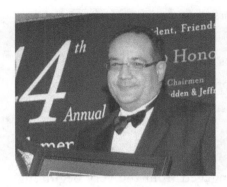

Cardiac and respiratory arrest and sudden cardiac death, are traumatic events for a patient, as well as for the family members and health care professionals that witnesses such an event. Despite all the advances in medicine, survival rates for a cardiac arrest are poor and a patient's best chance to survive is the initiation of rapid and adequate Basic Life Support (BLS) and CPR protocols.

BLS and CPR is a type of medical support using simple techniques to provide assistance. Any non-medical professional can acquire a basic CPR certification. However, BLS certification mandates a more in-depth education and training. These classes are intended to equip people with readily available and easy to utilize skills to aid in emergency first-aid needing quick and potentially life-saving intervention.

The task of taking the BLS and CPR course and certification exam can be intimidating for any student or healthcare provider as it reminds us that adequate and prompt institution of those techniques can be the only chance that a victim has to survive the arrest.

This book by authors Michele and Joseph Kunz is a wonderful tool that uses a more user-friendly approach. It is about learning. It is about keeping simple things simple and complicated concepts clear, concise, and (yes) simple too. They were able to use years of nursing and teaching experience to provide us with book and with a different format that any student will find innovative and easy to read. The whole process and base of the book is straightforward and is not the least intimidating.

It is about getting you from here to there (taking the course and passing it) without scaring you to death, boring you to tears or intimidating you. It's about increasing your knowledge, using some fun tricks, questions and answers, tips and notes. The question and answer section uses simple direct questions similar to the ones on the exam with concise answers. Also included, are sections on quick tips and notes that help the reader remember. There are several links to YouTube videos produced by the authors of this book. This is a tremendous help as the student can feel more at ease in mastering those important techniques.

Using this innovative fun format, the student remains engaged from the very beginning increasing his knowledge and self-confidence as he/she goes on reading. This method is also appealing as it simulates the clinical environment so well that it is easy to forget that you are mastering important concepts.

Although not a substitute for a comprehensive reference book, this textbook is ideal for first-time certification and for review of important concepts as well as for re-certification. It is equally useful for individuals who want to refresh their skills and update their knowledge. Of equal importance you will find that this approach is simply a fun way to learn and go on to passing the BLS and CPR course.

The authors Michele and Joseph are wonderful educators that have mastered the art of transmitting their vast knowledge into a wonderful book that's easy to read and to understand.

Thierry Duchatellier, MD
Section Chief of Cardiology
Mercy Medical Center, Rockville Centre, NY
St. Francis Medical Center, Rosyln, NY
Catholic Health Services of Long Island, NY

How This Book Will Help You Succeed

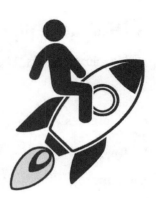

• This book will help you pass the BLS certification exam on your first attempt.

• We have created a video for every topic and article in this book, all available on YouTube.com/MicheleKunz.

• Lots of practical and usable information and advice about the BLS class and exam.

• 101 practice questions that cover every possible medical and nursing scenario and topic on the BLS certification exam.

• No confusing wrong answers to clutter your brain.

• Contains all the essential information for BLS exam success.

• This book, together with Michele's YouTube videos, will greatly reduce your test-taking anxiety.

• All information in this book has been updated to the current guidelines.

• Michele is always available for your email questions about this book, or any aspect of nursing or hospital work.

• Hot tips for surviving your first code.

• Hot tips to help you memorize lots of new information.

• Learn all of the biggest myths about the AED and CPR.

Who This Book Is Meant For

All healthcare providers and emergency responders such as:

• Physicians (MD's, DO's, DPM's)

• Nurses

• Paramedics

• Emergency Medical Technicians

• Respiratory Therapists

• Physical and Occupational Therapists

• Physician's Assistants

• Nurse Practitioners

• Residents and Fellows

• Technicians

• Aides and Healthcare Assistants

• Medical and Nursing Students

• Medical and Nursing Assistants

• Dentists

• Dental Assistants

• Police Officers

• All other allied health personnel

• Anyone who provides healthcare to patients in a wide variety of settings, including in-hospital and out-of-hospital

• For all certified, non-certified, and licensed healthcare professionals

Introduction

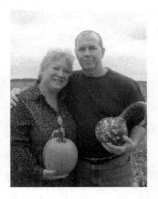

Our newly revised and enhanced book for 2017 that you now hold in your hands, *BLS Certification Exam Q & A With Explanations* will certainly help you pass any Basic Life Support Certification Course. As you look through the book, you will quickly see that this book's format is different from all other review and test preparation books.

This book is specifically geared toward healthcare students and new healthcare professionals that are preparing to take the BCLS/BLS/ CPR certification exam for the first time. This book will also give the seasoned healthcare professional lots of great review information as well as a way to update themselves on the latest research and guidelines.

Whichever certifying agency's program you are taking, either in a classroom or on the internet, this book will help you succeed in this course. In this book we give you all the essential information that you will need to successfully pass the certification course and exam on your first attempt.

Joe and I have been teaching this course to healthcare professionals and students since 1984. We know what works and what doesn't when it comes to helping our students be successful. Back then we had to develop almost all of the study materials for our students by ourselves because very little existed at the time. The *Zombie Notes Study Charts* were some of the first study aids we developed to help our students learn a large amount of information very quickly. We know that this format works very well because hundreds of thousands of healthcare professionals and students, in hospitals and colleges all over the world, have used this handy, no-nonsense chart to help them successfully pass the BLS and other certification exams.

Therefore, in order for you to be successful on the certification exam, and on the job, we expect you to memorize every bit of information contained within the *Zombie Notes Study Charts* and within this book. It is essential that you know this information by heart and can recall it at a moment's notice. This information is not only essential for the exam, but for your career, and the survival of your patients, as well.

You will find that the key to passing the certification exam and course lies in applying your knowledge through questions and answers, not rote memory alone. Memorization is simply the first step to learning and committing the information to your long-term memory. You will find that studying our book, and our *Zombie Notes Study Charts*, and watching our YouTube videos, all combine to make a very powerful study system, and a very productive and quick way to prepare yourself for success on the exam.

Therefore, in this book, we have created 101 practice questions that are designed to simulate actual exam conditions. The subject of BLS covers a lot of material. It is an interesting topic, and a working knowledge of the material is essential to do your job as a healthcare professional properly. In addition, we have tried to make studying for this exam as painless and as easy as possible. We have included all the essential information necessary for you to be successful on this exam. We have also included additional material to make studying this topic more fun and less painful.

We welcome your comments and suggestions. If you would like to offer a testimonial about how this book has helped you be successful, you will find more information about this at the end of the book.

We look forward to hearing from you. Good luck.
Joe and Michele Kunz
Long Island, New York

Part 1: About BLS

Notes

What Are BCLS, BLS, And CPR-Heartsaver Certification Courses All About?

Cardio-Pulmonary Resuscitation (CPR) is the basic term meaning to revive a person in cardiac and pulmonary arrest. This person's heart has stopped pumping blood and their breathing has stopped. There are no signs of breathing or response to the rescuer. If there is no breathing and no movement there probably isn't a heartbeat or pulse. The rescuer will call the emergency medical services (EMS) initially, begin CPR, and continue until help arrives.

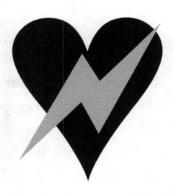

Basic Life Support (BLS) certification is a qualification demonstrating that someone has successfully completed a BLS course. This course reviews the risks for respiratory and cardiac arrest. Other topics such as stroke, first aide, and safety are often included in the certification program. The BLS program is required for most healthcare professionals (HCP) and must be taken at a minimum of every two years. Healthcare professionals are also required to learn and practice other more advanced skills.

These skills include using advanced airway and breathing devices. The CPR skills tested are chest compressions, ventilations, and relieving an obstruction in a choking victim. The bag - mask - ventilation (Ambu bag) is one device that replaces the "mouth-to-mouth" technique. HCP's are trained to perform CPR by themselves as well as with a second rescuer. The CPR procedures learned are different for adults, infants, and children. BLS for non-healthcare professionals focuses on one-person or one-rescuer. To successfully pass this course one must be able to perform the skills according to the instructor's expectations and pass a multiple-choice exam.

In all of the CPR courses, the participants will learn how to use an automated external defibrillator (AED). Once CPR has been started an AED can help save a life. The AED pads that are applied to the victim's chest, while CPR is in progress, can assess and determine the victim's heart (cardiac) rhythm, and prompt the rescuer to press the shock button.

Delivering an electrical shock with the AED can stop the heart that is quivering - and help restart it. The titles Basic Cardiac Life Support (BCLS) and Basic Life Support (BLS) can be used interchangeably, but now BLS is the most commonly used term.

The CPR Family and Friends/Heartsaver Program is a program that anyone can take – the general public as well as healthcare professionals. There are variations of this program that may include infant and children life-saving techniques. Always ask the instructor what is involved to prepare for class and what skills for which age groups. Healthcare professionals that can take the community-type programs Family and Friends/Heartsaver program as well. This might be necessary for a hospital or clinic-worker that cares for adults only, or they are not required to take the more advanced healthcare professional BLS Course. Again, the difference for the healthcare provider BCLS/BLS course is the advanced interventions using equipment and knowing the essential CPR skills for all age groups.

There are other programs that are available to healthcare professionals. These involve invasive techniques and the delivery of medications in order to resuscitate and stabilize the cardiac arrest victim after the basic life support has been started. The Emergency Medical Service (EMS) professionals are the first on the scene to apply these advanced life-saving skills. They will then transport the victim to a nearby medical center for care. These programs include Advanced Cardiac Life Support (ACLS), Pediatric Advance Life Support (PALS), Neonatal Resuscitation Program (NRP), and Trauma Certifications. The EMS personnel, hospital emergency room employees, and personnel from critical care units in the hospital are required to take programs like this and recertify every two years.

Finding a course to take should not be difficult. You can contact the American Heart Association (AHA), or American Red Cross (ARC) to find training centers in your neighborhood. Also, there are many ambulance and rescue services that offer CPR training to the community. Check the community library, community college, or local hospital for courses for the community or healthcare providers. There are "on-line" programs as well. These programs may not fulfill a requirement for healthcare professionals because these programs don't provide the "hands on" or "skills training" part of the course, that are usually required by a healthcare facility.

Upon successful completion of the skills and written exams you will receive a BLS certification card, which will be due for renewal in two years. Be very careful not to let your cards expire. To prepare for your BLS training there is reading material available. Ask the instructor for that ahead of time. You may also be expected to get down on your knees to perform the chest compressions for at least two minutes at a time. If you have any physical limitations be sure to tell your instructor so that accommodations can be made for you. You can also bring cushions for your knees. Gardening pads are great in this practice situation.

Once you are certified you may be interested in carrying your own personal pocket mask, so that direct mouth-to-mouth ventilations can be avoided. CPR science today recommends "high-quality, fast-and-hard" chest compressions with less emphasis on the initial mouth-to-mouth ventilations. The chest compressions are now considered so important that if the victim is in a cardiac arrest situation outside of the hospital – it is best to start compressions and the advanced airway interventions will begin when the EMS respond.

Course Length: 4 to 8 hours.

Intended Audience:
Healthcare providers, such as physicians, nurses, paramedics, emergency medical technicians, respiratory therapists, physical and occupational therapists, physician's assistants, residents or fellows, or medical or nursing students in training, aides, medical or nursing assistants, technicians, police officers, and other allied health personnel.

1. Information About The Certification Course

The Basic Life Support program is geared toward health professionals who work with victims and patients that may suddenly become ill and require CPR. The health professional may be dealing with the crisis as it starts, or continues the care as the patient progresses or continues to need advanced care. The course prepares one for recognizing and safely intervening in situations of medical emergencies such as respiratory arrest, stroke, and cardiac arrest.

If you have never taken a BLS Course before, there is ample study and reference materials, including study guides, pre-tests, and YouTube videos linked from MicheleKunz.com. Preparation and practice sessions, and having a comfort level with the topics, are key in passing BLS. You should dress in comfortable clothes because you will need to physically perform some of the skills and will need to get down on the floor to perform chest compressions. If you have any physical disabilities, discuss it with your instructor so that accommodations can be made to allow you to continue with the program. For example: the manikin can be placed on a table rather than the floor.

In the course you will be taking, there are written and skills testing of the automatic external defibrillators (AED's) and applying pads, use of simulation manikins, airway adjuncts such as pocket masks and bag-mask-ventilation devices. There will be individual and team practice sessions for all the skills, including one and two-rescuer adult, child, and infant, CPR skills. Practice will include positioning victims properly, assessing patient responsiveness, when to begin chest compressions, understanding CPR ratios, and how to relieve choking in conscious and unconscious victims. The BLS healthcare provider certification written exam is given during the program and an 84% or better is needed to pass.

The certification course requires preparation and participation in skills testing. If a student is unsuccessful in passing each part of the class, the instructor should reschedule for you to remediate or retake the course at another time.

2. Information About the Written Exam

The written exam has multiple-choice questions. It covers all the topics discussed from the written materials and practiced in the certification and re-certification classes. Usually, there is time allotted for remediation and review of the exam questions whenever necessary. To prepare for the written test it is necessary to take the practice pretest written exam. Bring any questions you have to class, or e-mail me any time at MKunz@MicheleKunz.com.

3. Information About the Lecture - Video Topics

The classroom/didactic session is a review of many topics in healthcare. The topics discussed include recognition of unresponsive victims and activation of emergency services, different age groups, and the science/evidence that applies to saving lives. Many health related topics such as MI, stroke, trauma, airway devices and using the automatic external defibrillator (AED) are also reviewed. Questions from the pre-test and the reading material are reviewed at this time as well. The instructor will play a video, which offers updated science explanations as well as demonstration sessions. The class also discusses the different types of rescuers, such as health professionals versus lay rescuers; how the Good Samaritan Law applies to us; and personal experiences of the instructor or students as well.

4. Information About the Skills Station Exam

The skills-station exam enables the participant to practice the hands-on skills until perfected. You will be expected to demonstrate proficiency in all the skills required to pass BCLS/BLS. Some skills will be practiced using hospital scenarios where the patient is in distress in his/her bed. Other scenarios may simulate victims in distress, choking, having symptoms of a stroke, and cardiac arrest in the home, restaurant, or street. The victim (manikin) will be on the floor, requiring immediate attention and/or CPR. You may also be asked to discuss the safety at the scene as well. Your safety is a priority in saving lives.

The manikins include adults, children, and infants. We will simulate conscious adult choking rescue on each other. The victims will become unconscious and the chest compressions to relieve the obstruction is begun on a manikin. The manikins can be on the floor or on a table surface to simulate life-like events.

Each participant is also required to properly position and apply AED pads to the victim's chest and follow the AED's prompts. You must be able to show the instructor that you can do this quickly, and without assistance.

Skills stations will assist you in identifying victims who are not breathing and have no palpable pulse. You will begin chest compressions utilizing the current guidelines. Cycles of CPR will be performed until the simulated cardiac arrest victim is resuscitated or EMS arrives and takes over. The team should then explicitly review their actions in a group debriefing to ensure that the best treatment was applied, and to consider team members and family emotions during and after the critical event.

10 Hot Tips for Passing the BLS and CPR Exam

Here is a guide to help you improve your chances of passing the exam for BLS – Basic Life Support. If you take the advice given here seriously, you will do very well on the exam. But you must allow yourself plenty of time to learn all of this material – especially if you are new to this. Watch our YouTube video on this topic at YouTube.com/MicheleKunz.

Tip # 1: Study And Memorize The *Zombie Notes Study Charts*
The *Zombie Notes* for BLS helps you study the need to knows and it is easy to take with you to study in your spare time. The study guide is not a replacement for the hands on practice and testing sessions that CPR class is known for. The *Zombie Notes* helps you memorize the important things that help you perform better. There are guidelines for all age groups with the most up to date information based on evidenced based practice and research.

Information on how to do correct techniques on infants, children (large and small) and adults are included. How to do one and two rescuer CPR, choking maneuvers for conscious and unconscious victims, AED operation and pads application, airway management and airway devices are explained.

Tip # 2: Read And Study The BLS Certification Manual
Your instructor should provide you with a textbook. It may be yours to keep or a loaner.

Tip # 3: Dress Comfortably And Be Prepared To Work On Your Knees
(explain to your instructor if this is not possible)

Tip # 4: Watch Michele's YouTube Videos On BLS, AED And Other Topics

Tip # 5: Take Practice Tests Over And Over Until You Get Them All Correct
There are questions on many topics, including age specific questions. Topics on the exam include AED use, safety at the scene of the victim, conscious and unconscious choking

victims, early defibrillation, landmarks for chest compressions, one and two rescuer CPR scenarios, initial assessments, infant techniques for two-rescuer CPR, depth and rate of compressions for all age groups, ventilations and advanced airways as well.

Tip # 6: Practice Doing Fast And Hard Compressions

Five (5) cycles of 30 compressions to 2 breaths can be practiced on a doll or cushion for 2 minutes, so you can perform high quality CPR at the class, know the landmarks for chest compressions for each age group, depth and recoil of compression, one hand, two hand and 2-thumb techniques for compressions.

Tip # 7: Review The Differences Between The Age Groups And The BLS Requirements For CPR

Review choking, AED pads, quick assessment for responsiveness, heart rates in infants that require initiation of chest compressions, breathing rates, pulse check sites, positioning of the airway, and recovery positions, starting CPR versus dialing 911 first, in infants and children, etc.

Tip # 8: Understand The Non-Trained "Hands Only" CPR Concept Versus Healthcare 30:2 CPR ratio

Mouth to mouth is not popular, nor recommended, in the initial stages of starting CPR. Consider purchasing your own face shield or pocket mask with a one-way valve.

Tip # 9: Read About The Related Topics

Read about the bag-mask ventilation (Ambu bag). Also, be sure to read about the pocket masks, positioning the victim's airway with or without suspected neck injury, and other airway adjuncts. First-aid is not usually included in the BLS program, but it may be needed for certain courses. Diagnosis such as myocardial infarction (heart attack) and stroke are life-threatening, and it is important to learn and recognize the symptoms.

Tip # 10: Participate In Class, And Ask And Answer Lots Of Questions

Speaking up and asking many questions helps you understand, memorize and will facilitate your classroom experience.

10 Hot Tips for Memorizing Information

Memorization is the fixing of information to your memory through sheer repetition. It is a necessary first step in learning. Memorization of essential terms and concepts of a difficult or new topic will provide a foundation for a deeper understanding that will follow with additional study. Michele and I teach thousands of healthcare professionals each year.

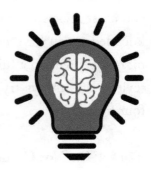

Everyone of them are expected to be able to quickly recall hundreds of essential dosages, formulas, and rules – all while under stress. Memorization, along with schooling, on-the-job training, in-house classes, and mandatory certifications, is an essential part of being a successful healthcare professional. Here is a list of our favorite ways to memorize a topic and its essential facts. Watch our YouTube video on this topic at YouTube.com/MicheleKunz.

Tip # 1: Break The Material Down Into Smaller Parts
Smaller bits of information will be much easier for your brain to hold onto. Make several lists. Work on memorizing these lists. Memorize a few facts, and them memorize a few more.

Tip # 2: Study In Short Periods Over A Long Period Of Time
Short burst of study, fifteen or thirty minutes at a time, are much better and more productive than sitting there and studying for sixty or ninety minutes. Whenever you are sitting somewhere, doctor's waiting room for example, take out your study cards and read them. These short busts of study periods can be very productive. Constantly doing this over many months is the surest way to get the information into your long-term memory.

Tip # 3: Review The Material Frequently

To get the new information from your short-term memory into your long-term memory you must review the material frequently. The more difficult the topic, and the less previous knowledge you have for a topic, the more frequently you must review the material. Some nights you will do a full study session of a subject. On the other nights you can do a quick review. But always try to touch upon that particular subject at least once every twenty-four hours.

Tip # 4: Do Not Cram

Cramming is usually useless. Learning a new or difficult topic takes time. Days, weeks, months, and years, not minutes. It takes a lot of time to process information properly.

Tip # 5: Use Mnemonics Devices And Catchy Puns And Phrases

Mnemonics are a great memory device to help your memorize difficult information. Here is one I created to remember the stages of shock: "Not His lucky CHARMS". Neurogenic, Hemmorhagic, Cardiogenic, Hypovolemic, Anaphylactic, Respiratory, Metabolic, Septic.

Tip # 6: Teach The Information To Another Person

This is probably one of the surest ways to force yourself to thoroughly learn a topic. Get a family member or friend to sit and let you explain a topic to them. Have them ask you questions and put you on the spot for an answer that is understandable. Don't just talk at the person. Really try to help them understand the subject.

Forcing yourself to explain the topic to another person will force your brain to put the topic into a format that your brain is comfortable with. This will get you past simple memorization, and you will start to really learn a subject.

Tip # 7: Use Various Study Materials

This simply means using different study materials, such as flash-cards, videos, study guides, etc. One night you might use the flash-cards and videos. The next night use the textbook and your notes. Another night use the flash-cards and a study guide, and so on.

Tip # 8: Leave The Radio/TV Off

You must minimize outside distractions. You must study the material as intensely as possible, with all of your concentration abilities, for short busts of time. Your brain can easily handle two or three tasks at the same time. But when studying, especially a new subject, is not the time to distracted by other things.

Tip # 9: Use A Study Chart/Cards

Make your own study chart or flash cards. This is a great way to help you recognize what information that you are having difficulty with.

Tip # 10: Study With A Friend

This will certainly make studying a difficult subject much more fun. It will also be a great way to test each other. It is also a way to make sure that you will study instead of watching television.

10 Hot Tips for Surviving Your First Code

Here is a guide to help you, the healthcare professional, start to become a productive participant in an in-hospital emergency (code blue). Watch our YouTube video on this topic at YouTube.com/MicheleKunz.

Tip # 1: Call For Help Prior To A Cardiopulmonary Arrest Occurs

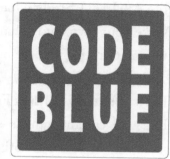

Yell down the hall for help, pick up the nearest phone, push the code button, and call the Rapid Response Team (RRT) or Medical Emergency Team (MET). Get help from your peers nearby as well as any code team or EMS that is on their way to help you. Call the team if you notice even subtle differences in the patient and their vital signs (including intractable pain). The RRT is to identify patient changes, call a team, and prevent clinical deterioration.

Tip # 2: Know The Emergency Number To Call

Post a sign with the number to call in an emergency and the name of your location and address if one would need to call EMS (911). In the hospital there may be a code number, a code button, intercom, RRT number, family RRT number. These numbers need to be memorized as well as clearly posted. When notifying the operator to page the team, be very clear with the location of the emergency, what type of emergency (cardiopulmonary arrest, stroke code, Rapid Response Team, security code, etc.).

Tip # 3: Stay Calm

When you know help is already on the way, you should be able to stay calm. Once you have called for help, the team and the equipment will be on the way. Getting yourself prepared for the worst emergency situation is also a great way to prepare your self. Decide what the worst thing that could happen to your patient could be, and decide what equipment you will most likely need. For example, if your patient is having trouble breathing, have an airway and bag-mask already in the room. If the IV is not running well, restart before an emergency occurs.

Tip # 4: Know How To Use Your Emergency Equipment

Before the emergency happens, you and your peers need to know where the emergency equipment is stored and how to use it properly. Know how to prepare the oxygen, suction and intubation equipment. Know what medications are in the code cart and what they are used for. This will help with your confidence in anticipating the patient's (and team) needs.

Tip # 5: Debriefing

Review the event afterwards to see what went well and what could have gone better. This includes the patient events and outcomes as well as how the team functioned together. Include the Pastoral Care or Social Work Department to help with emotional interventions for the family as well as meeting with staff members.

Tip # 6: Take Notes And Document Events

Document all vital signs (V/S), treatments, and decisions, during the event, with an exact timeline as best as possible during the event. You should keep your notes, especially if there could be a liability issue associated with the emergency situation.

Tip # 7: Certification And Review Courses

If you work in a procedural area of a hospital you probably should take a Basic Life Support (BLS) certification class. This class offers knowledge and skills regarding MI, stroke, chest compressions, automatic external defirillator (AED), and airway adjuncts.

Another great class to take is the Advanced Cardiac Life Support Course (ACLS). This certification class for health professionals is an intense course with cardiac arrhythmias, emergency treatments, medications and cardiopulmonary arrest as a priority topic. ACLS includes learning and testing stations, including a lengthy written exam.

Tip # 8: Be Willing To Help Others

If there is an emergency in a patient area that you are not currently assigned to, you should be quick to offer assistance. In this type of situation you can learn and gain more experience. Assist, watch, listen, and learn.

Tip # 9: Know Your Patient

It is important to have all the patient's history, blood work with any test results, and any recent changes in the patient's status. Review the patient's chart, listen carefully to the hand-off/report at the beginning of your shift. Do this before your hectic day begins. When the medical team arrives to the patient emergency they will have lots of questions about the patient. They will expect answers from you. Knowing these answers for the team allows for appropriate treatments, and perhaps faster and better patient outcomes.

Tip # 10: Post-Emergency or Code

The period after the code has ended is also a stressful time. It is great if the code is successful and the patient survives. However, the patient may now need a higher lever of care, and need to be transferred to a critical care area. Time is needed to document the events and the patient outcomes. Of course, this is the time that everyone thinks the code is "over", but the patient needs continuation of emergency care and supportive treatments.

You need to make sure that the practitioner stays with you and the patient, assisting you in ordering appropriate vasoactive infusions and medications while stabilizing the patient. If the patient does not survive the code, this is another time you don't want to be alone. You want another nurse, technician, or assistant to help with cleanup and preparing the body for a family viewing or transport to the morgue. Remember how you felt during this situation, and be there for your peers when it is their patient having the emergency situation.

Top 10 AED Myths

There are many automatic external defibrillators (AED) available in medical facilities as well as public places. Most of the public knows what an AED is - but have never had their hands on one or been trained on how to use one. And, because of this, many myths regarding AED use has developed. So, here is a list of the myths that Michele and I hear the most often from our healthcare students as well as the general public.

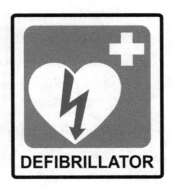

Myth # 1: AED's Are Difficult To Use

No. After you have called the emergency response team (Code "Blue" or 911) and you have begun CPR on a victim who appears pulseless and breathless, ask a bystander to get the AED. When an AED is available, simply turn it on and follow the AED's prompts. The AED's are easy to use and are highly accurate in determining if defibrillation (shock) is needed. The AED talks and prompts you through the correct and safe use of the pads. "Apply pads to patient's bare chest and plug in the connector". It is easier if one person can do the chest compressions while the other applies the AED pads. Anyone who has taken a CPR class learns about the AED and how to use it. Nothing difficult about it. If it is not working – just do chest compressions.

Myth # 2: If I Put The Pads On Wrong I Will Get Sued

No. The AED pads have pictures on the pads that explain where to apply the pads. If the pads aren't placed properly, the AED may ask you to correct their placement. If the AED cannot analyze or does not find a shockable rhythm, you will go back to high-quality chest compressions. Even if the victim is lying in snow, you can use an AED. The chest needs to be dry enough that the pads will stick. Hair may interfere with the pads abitlity to stick to the skin. Some AED's are equiped with a shaving razor. Otherwise, use a 2nd set ofpads to quikly pull off hair, in a fashion similiar to waxing.

We don't know of any lawsuits that have been brought against lay rescuers who attempt to provide CPR and use an AED. Generally speaking, our legal system provides nationwide Good Samaritan protection, exempting anyone who renders emergency treatment (outside the hospital setting) in an effort to save someone's life. Laws suits are usually focused around health clubs or similar institutions that have employees that did not have or use an AED at the time of a cardiac arrest.

Myth # 3: It Is Too Late To Deliver A Shock After 2 Minutes Of CPR

No, it is not too late. A rescuer must deliver, and continue to deliver, high quality CPR. When the AED does arrive and the pads are applied to the victim, the AED will determine if the victim is still in a shockable rhythm, and it will tell you to press the shock button. There is still a chance of survival.

Myth # 4: AED's Pads Are Not Interchangeable For Different Age Groups

Wrong. The AED pads are made for the specific age groups – one size for adults, and another for children, and still another for infants. But, of course, the most common age group for AED usage is the older adult. Adult pads can be used on the child 1 to 8 years old, and even on infants, if the correct size is not available. The pads will need to be placed on the front and back, avoiding the pads touching each other. Infant/child combo pads are available for use as well. Do not use smaller pads on adults, because it will not provide enough joules (defibrillation). In this case, continue applying chest compressions – high quality CPR. What is not interchangeable – is the brand or manufacturer of the pads. Use the brand of pads that is made for the AED that you have.

Myth # 5: The Chest Must Be Dry In Order For The AED Pads To Work

Wrong. Obviously the chest should be as dry as possible for the strongest and safest delivery of a shock. If possible, quickly dry off the chest, but do not delay defibrillation if the AED suggests a shock is required. A hairy chest can actually interefere with the pads sticking and giving an effective shock.

Myth # 6: Do Not Use The AED If The Victim Has A Pacemaker/Defibrillator, Medication Patch, Or Is In Contact With A Metal Surface

Wrong. If there is an apparent device under the skin where the pads would be placed, simply place the pads in another spot at least 2 inches away from the device. Remove any medication patch and dry the area. If you think the victim is being shocked by their own internal defibrillator, stand clear. Be prepared to start CPR and apply the AED pads as well. Call 911 as soon as possible. It has been proven that moving patients off of metal surfaces is unnecessary because there is very little risk to the CPR provider as long as they are not touching the victim when the shock is delivered.

Myth # 7: AED's Malfunction And Don't Give Enough Joules

Wrong. The number of AED malfunctions is very small compared to the number of the times AED's are used without a problem. AED's recognize shockable arrhythmias and can deliver up to 360 joules, based on the model. Data shows approximately 325,000 deaths annually due to sudden cardiac arrest (SCA) and that many of these lives could possibly be saved with the quick and proper use of and AED.

Myth # 8: Home AED's Do Not Save Lives

Approximately 80% of the deaths occur in the home, so it makes sense to have an AED in the home. However, family members often do not remember where the AED is located within their own home or within in their parent's home. Family members are also afraid to use it once the find the AED. They typically fear that they will use it incorrectly and harm their loved one. If the AED is used quickly and correctly, it can save a life. We must remember that AED's are very often used successfully in major public locations like shopping malls, airports, and casinos.

Myth # 9: I Need To Be A Healthcare Professional To Use The AED

Wrong. Certainly, if you are a health professional and use emergency equipment every day you would probably be comfortable using an AED - applying the pads and actually shocking someone. But the AED is so simple and straight forward to use that anyone in the general public can use successfully – even without taking a CPR certification class. But there are classes for the general public that include AED training.

Myth # 10: There Are No Resources For The Lifesaver In The Community

Wrong. There are plenty of life-saver and CPR classes in schools, libraries, community centers, and hospitals throughout America. There are also plenty of very good free videos on YouTube. The American Heart Association (AHA) sells a video with an inexpensive blow-up manikin to help a family practice their CPR skills. There are also applications for smart-phones that can help you call the 911, as well as guide you through the steps of CPR. There are also applications that alert CPR providers of emergency cardiac arrest calls that are close to their location.

Top 10 CPR Myths

Michele and I have been teaching CPR to healthcare professionals and students since 1984. We have seen the development, improvement, and wide-spread acceptance of CPR education over these years. Despite these advances, we still hear many myths about CPR every time we teach a class.

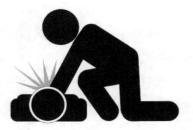

As healthcare professionals and students, we must not allow old information, nor the public's misperceptions and fears about CPR, nor Hollywood's unrealistic depiction of CPR, to affect our duty to provide high quality CPR to our patients and to the public. Therefore, in order to help dispel these myths, Michele and I have created this list of the most common CPR myths that we hear the most often from the healthcare professionals and students that we teach every day.

Myth # 1: CPR Must Include Mouth-To-Mouth Breathing
Wrong. Health professionals or first responders will initiate chest compressions immediately. The breaths should be done preferably with a bag mask, mouth to mask or mouth to mouth with a barrier device. If you do not have a barrier device or CPR face-mask, you can perform continuous chest compressions without ventilations until emergency services arrives. The American Heart Association has revised its recommendations and encouraged lay bystander rescuers to use "hands-only" CPR as an alternative to CPR with exchange of breaths.

Myth # 2: CPR Always Works
Wrong. Unfortunately, this is not true, and is a very common belief that has been perpetuated by Hollywood. The actual adult survival rate from out-of-hospital cardiac arrest is about 2 to 15%. Survival rates can increase up to 30% if an AED is used to deliver a shock. However, if the victim's heart stops and no one starts CPR immediately - then the victim's chance of survival is zero.

Myth # 3: I Could Get Sued If I Administer CPR In The Wrong Way Or Make A Mistake

Wrong. We have not read of any successful lawsuits that have been brought against lay rescuers or healthcare professionals who attempt to provide CPR. Generally speaking, our legal system provides nationwide Good Samaritan protection, exempting anyone who renders emergency treatment outside the hospital setting, with CPR in an effort to save someone's life. This includes lay rescuers and healthcare professionals. Lawsuits are usually focused around health clubs or similar institutions that have employees that did not have or use an AED at the time of a cardiac arrest. Generally, as long as lay rescuers and healthcare professionals do not waver too far from standard CPR procedure, they will most likely be protected.

Myth # 4: We Can Become Proficient In CPR With An On-Line Class

Wrong. While it is true that you can learn the steps of CPR from an on-line class, you most likely would not be able to perform high quality CPR on a real patient after taking a computer based CPR class. Hands-on practice, with the guidance of a certified instructor, is the key to developing muscle memory and proper techniques.

Myth # 5: We Can Save A Sudden Cardiac Arrest Victim With CPR Alone

Wrong. An AED/defibrillator can deliver shocks that will return the fibrillating heart to its normal rhythm. In most cases, CPR alone cannot revive a sudden cardiac arrest victim. CPR can delay death until a defibrillator delivers a lifesaving shock.

Myth # 6: A Patient Should Cough While Having A Heart Attack To Prevent The Heart Attack From Getting Worse

Wrong. This myth is what is known as 'Cough CPR'. Cough CPR was thought to speed up a very slow heart rate (bradycardia) and keep the patient conscious till emergency services arrived. It is probably a misinterpretation of the vagal maneuver. The vagal maneuver is used to help a patient stimulate the vagus nerve to slow down a fast heart rate.

Myth # 7: Cardiac Arrest Is The Same As A Heart Attack

Wrong. They are different conditions and are treated differently. Cardiac arrest is caused by an arrhythmia, dysrhythmia, electrolyte imbalance and trauma, which can lead to cardiac standstill, where the heart is not moving (asystole) or is fibrillating. A heart attack is a myocardial infarction, caused by a blocked coronary artery (acute coronary syndrome). Therefore, the term 'cardiac arrest' is not synonymous with 'heart attack'. A patient experiencing a heart attack may experience chest pain, nausea, vomiting, and become diaphoretic. However, a heart attack may ultimately lead to cardiac arrest depending on the severity of the blockage in the heart.

Myth # 8: Someone With More Experience Than Me Should Help The Victim. So I Shouldn't Help

Wrong. The key to surviving cardiac arrest is the immediate response of someone trained in CPR. A patient who collapses and does not immediately receive chest compressions has little or no chance of survival. If you know how to do chest compressions properly you should help immediately. Call for EMS initially then start chest compressions on the lower half of the breastbone.

Myth # 9: CPR Can Do More Harm Than Good

Wrong. When you are performing CPR it is on someone who has no heartbeat. Proper chest compressions, to be effective, must be fast and very hard. It is true that you may possibly break some of the victim's ribs while performing CPR. Once a victim is resuscitated injuries can be treated. Damaged ribs are worth the risk and much better than letting the victim die without attempting to give CPR. Ambulance personnel utilize a "thumper" device which uses a piston and plunger device, which is battery operated to do continuous chest compressions for lengthy period of times. Ribs may break with this device, however you can survive rib fractures.

Myth # 10: CPR Will Always Re-Start The Victim's Heart If They Are In Asystole

Wrong. CPR alone will not always re-start a heart that is not beating. The purpose of administering CPR is to push oxygenated blood to the victim's heart and vital organs. Continuing high quality CPR increases your chance of survival with a defibrillation when indicated. Emergency medications such as epinephrine may assist in getting the blood flow back into the heart and other vital organs (kidneys and brain).

4 Mechanical Devices That Can Help Improve CPR Delivery: An Introductory Guide

A variety of alternatives and adjuncts to conventional CPR have been developed with the aim of improving feedback during chest compressions, as well as improving cardiac output during the cardiac arrest. Conventional CPR consists of manual compressions and intermittent rescue breaths. But, over the years, various devices have been developed to enhance perfusion during resuscitation.

Here is a summary of the most common of these devices:

Mechanical Device # 1. Chest Compression Measurement and Feedback Devices

What Is It?

These chest compression measurement and feedback devices are usually hand-held, or defibrillator pads attached to a monitoring screen and sensors. They are able to measure and track the quality of chest compression performance in real-time. Some of these devices can simultaneously measure the depth, rate, and force of chest compressions.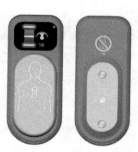

How Does It Improve CPR Delivery?

When this device is used during CPR training, it can be attached to a computer that can provide immediate data feedback on compression depth, rate, and force. It can also provide a downloadable summary of CPR performance for the entire duration of the event for peer review.

It will also give you immediate feedback and encourage you to perform to meet the expectations of:

1. Ideal depth of 2 to 2-1/2 inches for adults

2. Requirement of 100 to 125 lbs. of downward force

3. At the rate of at 100 – 120 chest compressions per minute, with full recoil.

This device can improve CPR delivery initially, if used during the CPR classroom training program. Some manikins offer clicking sounds and lights when compressing hard enough. There newer devices may have verbal prompts, measure rate, and depth and a way to analyze the compressor's performance. This device helps the CPR student get a more realistic feel for what is physically needed to provide effective chest compressions. During a real cardiac arrest, it may assist the compressor/healthcare professional, in giving the victim the best chance for survival.

Mechanical Device # 2. Automatic Chest Compression Machine (Thumper, Lucas Machines)

What Is It?
The automatic chest compression machine is a mechanical hands-free CPR device capable of delivering automated and continuous chest compressions to a patient in cardiac arrest. Once this device is set-up on the patient, it can provide high-quality chest compressions consistently and for a long period of time, depending on the power supply.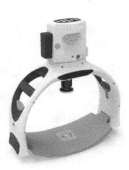

How Does It Work?
The frame of this machine is placed under the victim's back and over the chest. It then utilizes a piston device that sits atop of the patient's chest. The patient's arms are then fastened to the device to ease transport of the patient. CPR can then be delivered even if the patient is being transported down a flight of stairs.

How Does It Improve CPR Delivery?
It improves CPR delivery because the compressions that it delivers provides consistent depth and speed. Once it is set up properly, it allows the rescuers to concern themselves with other lifesaving tasks. This device is beneficial when there is a need for high-quality chest compressions, for a long time.

Mechanical Device # 3. Capnography Monitor

What Is It?

Waveform capnography is the continuous, noninvasive measurement and graph/numerical display of partial end-tidal carbon dioxide (PETCO2). The patient or victim has a nasal device, similar to the nasal oxygen tubing. The victim can also receive oxygen through this device. When the victim or patient exhales, the carbon dioxide is measured. The capnography monitor is a portable or bedside device used to monitor a patient's respiratory status. This monitor delivers

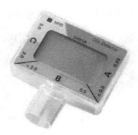

Yellow, yes; Purple, poor.

real-time, continuous monitoring of the patient's respiratory status by measuring PETCO2. It can also be attached to the intubated patient's endotracheal tube on the ambulance, in the OR, procedural areas, or critical care areas. If the patient were to stop breathing the capnography alarm would alert the healthcare provider within 30seconds.

The 2015 AHA Guidelines for ACLS recommend using quantitative waveform capnography in intubated patients during CPR. Waveform capnography allows healthcare professionals to monitor CPR quality, optimize chest compressions, and detect return of spontaneous circulation (ROSC) during chest compressions. These devices are used routinely on ambulances, in endoscopy centers, operating rooms, diagnostic sleep centers, ambulatory surgical centers, and critical care settings.

How Does It Improve CPR Delivery?

During CPR, capnography can help the team determine if chest compressions are effective. If pressing deep enough on the chest, exhaled carbon dioxide can be measured. Capnography or partial end-tidal CO2 (PETCO2) should be greater than 10mmHg, which means you are doing adequate, deep and hard compressions. If the number is

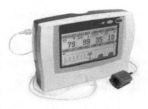

below 10, the compressions need to be deeper. If normal CO2 (35 to 40 mm Hg) is displayed on the monitor, this would be an indication of return of spontaneous circulation (ROSC).

Mechanical Device # 4. Portable Automated External Defibrillator (AED) Device

What Is It?

These can be very useful, especially since they typically do not require special medical training. They are usually found in public places, such as offices, airports, train stations, gyms, and shopping centers. They are only used if one has already started chest compressions.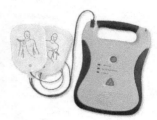

The AED will expressly tell you exactly what to do as soon as it is turned on. When the AED is turned on, it will tell the rescuer to apply pads to the victim's bare chest, it will be analyzing the cardiac rhythm, tells the rescuer to stand clear, and then will charge itself and tell you to deliver a shock if appropriate.

How Does It Improve CPR Delivery?

The AED doesn't necessarily improve compression delivery, but compressions can enhance the chances of the electrical shock (defibrillation) working. The AED will tell you when to stop or return to compressions.

Conclusion

Overall, the easiest and fastest way to deliver high-quality CPR is manually. But measurement devices can help improve training healthcare professionals in proper and effective techniques by giving real-time feedback. And the mechanical devices such as the Thumper can help improve patient outcomes when used in the field and in the hospital by keeping the compressions at a consistent depth and rate. And the AED can help improve CPR by delivering the shock at the most appropriate time.

Notes

Part 2:
The Questions

Notes

Certification Exam Practice Questions For BLS

1. How do you know if your ventilations are adequate, whether it is mouth to mask, bag mask ventilations, or mouth-to-mouth breaths?

a. You can see the stomach rising with each breath

b. You can hear the air coming out of the victim's nose

c. The chest rises with each breath you administer

d. There is no stomach or chest movement while administering the breaths

2. What is the definition of the term "to recoil" completely after each chest compression?

a. Keeping the chest pushed down approximately 1 inch between compressions

b. Keeping the chest pushed down approximately 2 to 2-1/2 inches between compressions

c. Taking your weight off your hands and allow the chest to come back to its normal position

d. The sound of breaking ribs after each completion

3. In BLS, two minutes is considered 5 cycles. Within one cycle what is the ratio of compressions to ventilations in one-rescuer CPR (all ages)?

a. 100 compressions to 2 breaths

b. 30 compressions to 2 breaths

c. 100 compressions to 1 breath

d. 30 compressions to 1 breath

4. When a victim has fallen or there is neck trauma suspected, how does the rescuer open the victim's airway?

a. Do not touch them and call 911

b. Use the head tilt/chin lift

c. Use the tongue lift/finger sweep

d. Use the modified jaw thrust maneuver

5. How fast is the rate of compressions per minute for victims of any age?

a. Up to 25 compressions per minute

b. At least 100 to 120 compressions per minute

c. 500 compressions per minute

d. 1,000 compressions per minute

6. What are the signs of adequate breathing from the victim? Looking at the chest is one of the signs. What other signs do you assess for?

a. Arterial Blood Gas

b. Feeling the skin temperature

c. Listening at the victim's mouth

d. Listen for gas movement in the abdomen

7. What is the best way for a rescuer to know that a rescue breath for an infant victim is effective?

a. The infant vomits

b. A wheeze is heard

c. The chest rises

d. The rescuer can see the infant's hair blowing with the breaths

8. When a victim is barely breathing (agonal gasps), but has a pulse, and someone has called the emergency medical system (EMS), what should you do?

a. Check the victim's pulse for a minute

b. Open the victim's eye and look for pupillary response

c. Open the airway, give 2 breaths, and then 1 breath every 5 to 6 seconds

d. Call EMS again

9. When should a rescuer begin chest compressions with breaths (CPR) for an adult?

a. The adult is responding but is complaining of heartburn

b. The adult is not responsive but is breathing

c. The adult is not responding, not breathing, and you cannot feel a pulse

d. The adult has a fast pulse and trouble breathing

10. How is CPR done on infants ages birth to 1 year old when there are two healthcare providers?

a. One rescuer gives cycles of 30 compressions and 2 breaths while the second rescuer waits 2 minutes for his turn

b. You stop giving CPR while the second rescuer checks the victim's pulse, and then you continue with cycles of 30 compressions and 2 breaths

c. Cycles of 15 compressions and 2 breaths with one rescuer giving chest compressions and the other giving the breaths

d. Three rescuers together using the 2-thumb encircling hands technique.

11. How is CPR done on infants ages birth to 1-year-old when there is one healthcare provider?

a. One rescuer gives cycles of 30 compressions and 2 breaths

b. One rescuer cannot do CPR on an infant alone CPR

c. Cycles of 15 compressions and 2 breaths

d. Cycles of 25 compressions to 2 breaths using the 2-thumb encircling hands technique

12. What is the ratio and method for one-rescuer CPR on children ages 1 to 12-years-old?

a. Ratio is 30 compressions to 2 breaths using one or two hands

b. Ratio is 15 compressions to 2 using two fingers

c. Ratio is 100 compressions to 2 breaths

d. Three rescuers together using the 2-thumb encircling hands technique

13. Why is it important to do fast and hard CPR and provide early defibrillation to an adult?

a. The CPR is not as important as the defibrillation

b. The most effective treatment for sudden cardiac arrest is CPR alone

c. The most effective treatment for sudden cardiac arrest is defibrillation alone

d. Successful defibrillation relies on the high quality CPR given continuously up to that time

14. What is the first thing to be done when the automatic external defibrillator (AED) is brought to the side of a cardiac arrest victim?

a. Shave the victim's chest, and press the SHOCK button

b. Turn on the AED, apply pads to the victim's chest

c. Power on the AED, and press SHOCK button immediately

d. Turn on the AED, check the pulse just prior to applying the pads

15. At what time during the cardiac arrest rescue are the automatic external defirillator (AED) pads applied?

a. Pads are applied after 10 minutes of CPR

b. As soon as the EMS arrive at the scene

c. Pads are applied in the emergency department

d. The AED pads are applied as soon as they are made available

16. What could happen if you or someone in the team or crowd is touching the victim while the AED is delivering a shock?

a. The AED will sense that there is a dangerous situation

b. The AED will recognize the responders heart rhythm

c. The AED could shock you while it is shocking the victim

d. The AED will ask you to reapply the pads

17. When using an AED, the AED says "no shock advised", what should you do next?

a. Disconnect and plug in the pads to re-start the AED again

b. Remove the pads from the victim's chest and wait for the EMS to arrive

c. Remove the pads from the victim's chest and continue CPR

d. Leave the pads on the victim's chest and continue with compressions

18. An adult victim standing next to you has an obstructed airway, how will you help this choking victim?

a. Start chest compressions immediately

b. Perform abdominal thrusts until the obstruction is relieved or victim is unconscious

c. Give 5 back slaps, followed by breaths until they go in

d. Give breaths, repositioning the airway after each breath

19. The abdominal thrusts are not working to relieve an obstructed airway. The victim becomes unconscious and you slide him/her onto their back. The waiter has already called 911. What should you do next?

a. Perform a jaw thrust and attempt to deliver breaths

b. Continue the abdominal thrusts until the object comes out

c. Begin chest compressions immediately, always looking for the object to come out

d. Give mouth to mouth for 2 minutes, until you can get the air through

20. You begin the steps of CPR on an infant you find who is not responding at a daycare center. When should you call the emergency medical system (EMS)?

a. After you complete 20 cycles of CPR

b. After you check the infant's pulse

c. After all attempts to resuscitate fail

d. Call (or have someone call) EMS as soon as you find the unconscious infant

21. There are two health professionals performing BLS on an infant. What is the correct ratio for chest compressions and ventilations for two-rescuer child CPR?

a. 15 compressions to 2 breaths

b. 30 compressions to 2 breaths

c. 100 compressions to 2 breaths

d. 5 compressions to 2 breaths

22. How do you relieve choking in conscious children and adults?

a. Cycles of 5 back slaps, and 5 chest compressions, until the child is unconscious

b. Perform abdominal thrusts until the object comes out, or the victim becomes unconscious

c. Give breaths, until the air goes in

d. Wait till they become unconscious and begin chest compressions.

23. Why are chest compressions done fast, hard, and with minimal interruptions to victims of any age?

a. Interrupting chest compressions is the only chance the rescuer has to rest

b. Minimizing interruptions leads to improved blood flow and a higher rate of survival

c. Only cardiologists are allowed to have interruptions in their chest compressions

d. The faster and harder compressions are done, the more calories the rescuer will burn

24. A pulseless child is receiving CPR, and an AED is brought to the scene. There aren't any pediatric pads available. Pediatric pads have an attenuator that dramatically reduce the joules delivered. At this time can you use the adult pads on the child?

a. Yes, but make sure the pads do not touch each other

b. No, you can only use pediatric AED pads

c. Yes, but use only one adult pad

d. Children do not require AED or defibrillation pads - ever

25. **When the paramedic team arrives, they successfully insert an endotracheal tube into the victim's airway. The recommended rate for ventilations through the advanced airway is slower. What is the ventilatory rate for this victim?**
a. Two breaths every 5 to 6 seconds
b. Two breaths every 6 to 8 seconds
c. One breath every 5 to 6 seconds
d. One breath every 6 to 8 seconds

26. **You are holding the choking infant in your arms. What is the most effective way to remove the obstructed object in the conscious/awake infant?**
a. Perform abdominal thrusts
b. Cycles of 5 backslaps, and 5 chest compressions, until the infant becomes
   unconscious, then begin CPR
c. Give breaths, until the air goes in
d. Give the baby a bottle of water to drink

27. **How often should the rescuers switch during 2-rescuer adult CPR?**
a. Every 30 minutes
b. Every 15 cycles of 30 compressions to 2 breaths
c. Every 10 cycles of 30 compressions to 2 breaths
d. Every 5 cycles of 30 compressions to 2 breaths

28. **CPR should be started prior to the AED application and initiated immediately after . . . ?**
a. A pulse check
b. Two (2) quick breaths
c. The defibrillation is delivered
d. Emergency medical services arrive

29. When compressing the infant's chest the rescuer must compress the chest how many inches?

a. 1-1/2 inches

b. 2 inches

c. 2-1/2 inches

d. 3 inches

30. How long should a rescuer take when checking a victim's responsiveness, breathing and pulse?

a. The rescuer should check for response, breathing, and pulse, within 10 seconds

b. The rescuer should not check for breathing or pulse, just start CPR

c. The rescuer should check breathing and pulse for 10 minutes

d. The rescuer should check for a pulse only if the victim is under 50 years old

31. The AED can be obtained and turned on by . . . ?

a. Paramedics only

b. Only first responders with proper training

c. Anyone regardless of their training

d. All of the above

32. The automatic external defirillator (AED) can save a life by . . . ?

a. Recognizing pulseless ventricular rhythms

b. Advising rescuers to continue chest compressions

c. Advising the rescuers a defibrillation is needed

d. All of the above

33. Practicing and testing with the AED and pads is mandatory in CPR/BLS courses because . . . ?

a. Pads can be reused many times on victims/patients

b. Practice prepares a rescuer for the real situation

c. Coordinated team efforts with the AED and compressions lead to greater success

d. Both b and c

34. The best place to check a pulse on an infants is . . . ?

a. The carotid artery

b. The femoral artery

c. The brachial artery

d. The temporal artery

35. The best place to check a pulse on a child is . . . ?

a. The carotid artery

b. The femoral artery

c. The brachial artery

d. The temporal artery

36. The best place to check a pulse on an adult is . . . ?

a. The carotid artery

b. The femoral artery

c. The brachial artery

d. The temporal artery

37. The child is considered to be between the ages of 1-year and 12-years-of-age. Ages 1 through 8 are considered "small" children. What is the technique for chest compressions for the small child?

a. Two hands

b. The heel of one hand

c. Two finger technique

d. None of the above

38. How are chest compressions (2 inches deep) performed on a large child ages 8 to 12?

a. Two hands

b. The heel of one hand

c. Two finger technique

d. None of the above

39. When opening the airway of an unconscious infant victim, the technique used is often called . . . ?

a. The sniffing position

b. Pinching the nose

c. Tilt head forward

d. Head tilt, chin lift, or jaw thrust

40. When assessing the victim for responsiveness, you should . . . ?

a. Watch for his chest rise and fall

b. Listen for exhaled air by the victim's mouth and nose

c. Check the pulse for 10 seconds.

d. All of the above

41. If the infant/child is unresponsive and you are alone, you should . . . ?

a. Complete 5 to 10 cycles of CPR

b. Knock on neighbors door to get help

c. Begin CAB of CPR and activate the emergency medical services immediately

d. Give the infant/child five back slaps and 5 chest compressions

42. When ventilating a child with a bag mask device . . . ?

a. Breath as quick as you possibly can

b. Ventilate to see rise and fall of the chest

c. Ventilate at the rate of 3 breaths per minute

d. All of the above

43. Chest compressions on an infant is performed at what depth?

a. 1/2 inch deep, above the nipple line

b. 1 inch deep, at the nipple line

c. 1-1/2 inches deep, one finger breath below the nipple line

d. 2 inches deep, nipple line

44. Which is the most effective method of chest compressions in two-rescuer CPR for the infant victim?

a. The two-knuckle technique

b. The heel-of-one-hand technique

c. Two-hand technique

d. The two-thumb technique

45. Chest compressions on a child are at what depth?

a. 1/2 inch deep

b. 1 inch deep

c. 1-1/2 inches deep

d. 2 inches deep

46. Chest compressions on an adult are at what depth?

a. 1/2 inch deep

b. 1 inch deep

c. 1-1/2 inches deep

d. 2 to 2 1/2 inches deep

47. When performing the abdominal thrusts on a conscious choking child or adult, how do you know you are doing it successfully?

a. The choking victim becomes unconscious

b. The choking victim begins to cough and breath on their own

c. Pulling your fist inward and upward from the victims waistline

d. Both b and c

48. When the conscious choking victim becomes unconscious and is gently placed on the ground, the rescuer must . . . ?

a. Call the emergency medical services and immediately begin chest compressions and ventilations (30:2)

b. Call the emergency medical services and wait for them to come

c. Perform a finger sweep until the victim vomits

d. Turn the victim on their side hoping the victim will vomit

49. When doing chest compressions at the victim's side and you are alone, which ventilation device or method would be the most difficult to perform alone and take the most time to use?

a. Mouth to mouth ventilation

b. Mouth to mask ventilation

c. Bag-mask ventilation

d. Ventilations are not required during one rescuer CPR

50. Before approaching a victim in an unfamiliar environment the rescuer must . . . ?

a. Call the emergency medical services

b. Ensure that area is safe to approach

c. Phone a friend for advice

d. Both a and b

51. If the AED is not working properly, what should be done immediately?

a. Call the manufacturer immediately

b. Take the time to check all connections

c. Immediately start chest compressions

d. None of the above

52. The Basic Life Support (BLS) Certification card needs renewal every . . . ?

a. 6 months

b. 1 year

c. 2 years

d. 5 years

53. An infant appears to be choking, what are the signs and symptoms of an infant choking?

a. The infant will be absolutely silent

b. The infant will be able to pull the object out

c. The infant will make high pitch sounds and may turn bluish

d. The infant will remain pink

54. What is the procedure to relieve an obstruction in the conscious choking infant?

a. Perform abdominal thrusts

b. Perform finger sweeps

c. Perform chest compressions

d. Perform 5 back slaps and 5 chest compressions

55. What are the signs and symptoms of a child choking?

a. The child will be absolutely silent

b. The child will continue to play

c. The child can make high pitch sounds or be silent

d. The child will remain pink

56. What is the procedure to relieve an obstructed airway in a conscious choking child?

a. Perform abdominal thrusts

b. Perform finger sweeps

c. Perform chest compressions

d. Perform 5 back slaps and 5 chest compressions

57. An adult appears to be choking, what are the signs and symptoms of an adult choking?

a. The adult will be silent, and may raise their arms to their neck

b. The adult will be able to pull the object out

c. The adult will make high pitch sounds

d. The adult will remain pink

58. What is the procedure to relieve an obstructed airway in a conscious choking adult?

a. Perform abdominal thrusts

b. Perform finger sweeps

c. Perform chest compressions

d. Perform 5 back slaps and 5 chest compressions

59. If a choking victim of any age becomes unconscious, what should the rescuer do?

a. Perform abdominal thrusts

b. Call 911 (EMS) and begin chest compressions

c. Hyperventilate the victim

d. Turn the victim on the side

60. You have cleared the airway on an unconscious choking victim, doing high quality chest compressions. You already called 911 (EMS). What should you do now?

a. Check for breathing and pulse

b. Leave the victim to wash your hands

c. Lie the victim on his stomach

d. Check the pockets for a family contact phone number

61. You have cleared the airway on an unconscious choking victim. There is a pulse and the victim is breathing. What should you do now?

a. Turn the victim on the side - the recovery/rescue position

b. Begin chest compressions with ventilations

c. Begin chest compressions without ventilations

d. Begin ventilations without compressions

62. What equipment would a rescuer need to perform Basic Life Support?

a. Advanced airway equipment

b. A pocket mask/face shield and an AED

c. A medication cart

d. An intraosseous drill

63. The AED is an . . . ?

a. Agitated Elevated Diaphragm

b. Automatic External Defibrillator

c. Automatic Estimated Delivery

d. Atropine, Epinephrine, Diazepam

64. The AED is equipped with defibrillator pads. What sizes are usually available in the hospital setting?

a. Adult pads only

b. Adult and child pads are used interchangeably

c. Cut the adult pads to make pediatric or infant pads

d. Adult, child, and infant size pads are available

65. What if you only have pediatric pads available? Can you use them on an adult?

a. No, the energy is not high enough, begin chest compressions

b. Yes, use any size pad you have on the adult

c. Yes, use the pediatric pads if it is a smaller adult

d. Yes, place the pads closer to the heart

66. Are all AED pad connectors universal and fit into every AED or defibrillator cable?

a. Yes, all pads are compatible to any manufacturers connectors

b. No, pads and connectors are not universal

c. Yes, if they are made in the United States

d. Yes, there is only one manufacturer making AED pads

67. What is the compression depth for an infant of 8-months-old?

a. 2 inches deep

b. 1 inch deep

c. 1-1/2 inches deep

d. 1/2 inch deep

68. Two health professionals are doing CPR on an infant. One rescuer is ventilating, and the other is compressing. Which technique is used for two-rescuer CPR for the infant victim?

a. The two-thumb compression technique, with the fingers around the infants back

b. The heel-of-one-hand technique, compressing 2 inches deep

c. Two-hand technique, compressing 1 inch deep

d. Back blows and chest compressions

69. What is the depth of chest compressions for a child, ages 1 to 12-years-old?

a. 1/2 inch deep

b. 1 inch deep

c. 1-1/2 inches deep

d. 2 inches deep

70. What is the depth of chest compressions on an adult victim with no pulse?

a. 1/2 inch deep

b. 1 inch deep

c. 1-1/2 inches deep

d. 2 to 2-1/2 inches deep

71. What is the ratio of compressions to ventilations for one or two-rescuer adult CPR?

a. 30 compressions : 2 breaths (30:2)

b. 15 compressions : 1 breath (15:1)

c. 15 compressions : 2 breaths (15:2)

d. 5 compressions : 2 breaths (5:2)

72. What is the ratio of compressions to ventilations for one-rescuer infant or child CPR?

a. 15 compressions : 1 breath (15:1)

b. 15 compressions : 2 breaths (15:2)

c. 30 compressions : 2 breaths (30:2)

d. 5 compressions : 2 breaths (5:2)

73. What is the ratio of compressions to ventilations for two-rescuer infant or child CPR?

a. 3 compressions : 1 breath (3:1)

b. 5 compressions : 2 breaths (5:2)

c. 15 compressions : 2 breaths (15:2)

d. 30 compressions : 2 breaths (30:2)

74. What is the placement position of the two AED pads for an effective defibrillation?

a. Left and right arms

b. On both sides of the umbilicus

c. Left side at the lower rib cage, and below the right clavicle

d. Place both pads on the back

75. If the infant victim requires airway support and ventilation using the bag-mask, how will you know if the breaths are adequate?

a. There will be a high pitched sound with adequate breaths

b. There will be a capillary refill of 10 seconds with adequate breaths

c. There will be rise and fall of the abdomen with adequate breaths

d. There will be rise and fall of the chest with adequate breaths

76. What is the proper ventilation rate for infant and child rescue-breathing?

a. Two breaths every 10 seconds

b. Two breaths every 3 to 5 seconds

c. One breath every 10 seconds

d. One breath every 3 to 5 seconds

77. When compressing the chest of an adult, where is the correct placement of your hands?

a. One hand in the center of the chest

b. Two hands on the lower one-half of the sternum/breastbone

c. Two hands, 2 finger breaths above the nipple line

d. Two hands, at the level of the umbilicus

78. Mechanical devices that assist and improve CPR delivery are . . . ?

a. Chest compression measurement and feedback device

b. Automatic chest compression (thumper) machine

c. Capnograph device (measurement of exhaled CO_2)

d. All of the above

79. When a victim has an occluded airway, what part of the anatomy is obstructed?

a. The mouth and lower intestine

b. The esophagus and umbilicus

c. The vocal cords and trachea

d. The Eustachian tubes and the cochlear

80. The abdominal thrust is not working to relieve the obstructed airway in the victim. Just prior to the victim becoming unconscious, what other lifesaving maneuvers might work?

a. Chest thrust, from behind the choking victim

b. Back slaps

c. Raising the arms above the head

d. Both a and b

81. If you are alone and an adult needs resuscitation what should you do first?

a. Do 5 minutes high quality CPR

b. Begin backslaps

c. Bundle up the baby and get to your car

d. Phone emergency medical services (911)

82. A choking child becomes unconscious and is on the floor. What should you do?

a. Continue with abdominal thrusts

b. Begin backslaps

c. Drive the victim to the hospital in your car

d. Phone emergency services (911) and begin chest compressions

83. What is the survival rate for CPR?

a. The adult survival rate from out-of-hospital cardiac arrest is about 2 to 15%

b. The survival rate from out-of-hospital cardiac arrest is 80 to 90%

c. The survival rate from out-of-hospital cardiac arrest has not been determined

d. The adult survival rate from out-of-hospital cardiac arrest is 0%

84. What will increase the survival rate for cardiac arrest victims?

a. Lying the patient in ice-cold water

b. Using the automatic external defibrillator (AED)

c. Delivering 100% oxygen immediately

d. Delivering compressions at the rate of 60 to 80 beats per minute

85. Why is debriefing important after a team intervention occurs?

a. Allows the team to have a coffee break on a busy day

b. Time for removal of the victim/patients clothes for a good exam

c. Review the event afterwards to see what went well and what could have gone better

d. Gives the nurse time to enter all the information into the electronic medical record

86. Who is required to take the BLS program for healthcare providers?

a. All high school students

b. Paramedics, physicians, and nurses

c. All teachers

d. Spouses of patients with cardiac disease

87. A 78-year-old woman tells you, "I think I am having a stroke". What are the signs and symptoms you are looking for?

a. Weakness and numbness on one side of her body

b. Slurred speech

c. Facial droop

d. All of the above

88. What is universal precautions, and what is needed to perform CPR?

a. Universal precautions protect the victim from being identified and none is needed with CPR

b. Universal precautions protect you in case you are late for work, and you need that - so not to get fired

c. Universal precautions protect from infectious diseases, and you need gloves and a pocket mask

d. All of the above

89. You are doing compressions on an adult victim. The automatic external defibrillator (AED) only has pediatric pads. What are you doing next?

a. Use the pediatric pads if it is all you have

b. Continue chest compressions

c. Turn the AED off then on again, so it will reanalyze

d. Place both pediatric pads over the victim's heart on the left side

90. You are caring for a 6-month-old infant, whose condition has been deteriorating. When would you begin chest compressions on an infant?

a. Begin chest compressions on the infant if the heart rate is less than 60 beats per minute

b. Begin chest compressions if the heart rate is more than 60

c. Begin chest compressions if the heart rate is less than 100

d. Begin chest compressions only when there is no pulse

91. How often should you check a pulse on adults, infants and children, once CPR has been initiated?

a. A pulse should be checked every 10 seconds

b. A pulse should be checked every 10 minutes

c. A pulse should be checked with every two-minute CPR switch

d. It is not necessary to check the pulse

92. What is the typical cause of cardiac arrest in children?

a. Gunshot wounds are the number one cause of death

b. Progressive deterioration in respiratory function is the typical cause of cardiac arrest

c. Natural causes of death is the usual cause of cardiac arrest

d. Infectious disease is the number one cause of cardiac arrest

93. Why is the two-thumb technique more effective for infant CPR?

a. Two-thumb technique is not effective in infant CPR

b. The two-thumb technique is used to compress the umbilicus

c. The two-thumb technique produces better blood flow, and consistent depth and artificial blood pressure (perfusion)

d. The two-thumb technique allows compressions and no need for ventilations

94. What are the implications of a victim lying on wet ground, when applying the automatic external defibrillator (AED)?

a. The victim can be lying in a wet area if it is impossible to move the victim

b. The victim's chest should be as dry as possible

c. Water will enhance the defibrillation through the victim's chest

d. Both a and b

95. Why is it important to avoid applying the automatic external defibrillator (AED) pads on top of medicated patches?

a. There is no difference in the defibrillation if delivered through a medicated patch

b. The medicated patches can cause a large explosion on the chest if the AED delivers a shock

c. The medicated patch will double the amount of joules delivered to the victim

d. The medicated patch can actually cause burns on the skin and prevent the joules being delivered to the victim

96. The victim is pulseless and breathless. Emergency services are on their way. You begin chest compressions. Another rescuer asks if they can help. What will you tell the second rescuer to do?

a. The second rescuer should get the nearest AED and apply the pads

b. The second rescuer should dial 911 again

c. The second rescuer should begin the ventilations

d. Both a and c

97. The Good Samaritan Law are laws or acts offering legal protection to people who give reasonable assistance to those who are injured, ill, in peril, or otherwise incapacitated outside the hospital setting. This law applies to . . . ?

a. Physician and nurses

b. Therapist or registered physician's assistant

c. The general public

d. All of the above

98. A myocardial infarction (heart attack) may ultimately lead to cardiac arrest depending on the severity of the blockage in the heart. What are the signs and symptoms of a heart attack?

a. Chest pain

b. Nausea, vomiting and diaphoresis (sweating)

c. Blurred vision

d. Both a and b

99. When a victim has chest pain and you already have called the Emergency Medical Services (911), what else can you do while waiting for the ambulance?

a. Leave the victim and wait outside for the ambulance

b. See if the victim can chew a regular aspirin

c. Have the victim walk down the stairs to get closer to the ambulance

d. Offer the victim coffee to stimulate the heart rate

100. Stroke is a disease of physical complications including weakness and paralysis. What are the signs and symptoms of stroke?

a. Slurred speech

b. Headache and sensory loss

c. Vision changes

d. All of the above

101. When a victim has the signs and symptoms of stroke what is the best immediate action to take?

a. Have the victim drink a large bottle of water

b. Take two (2) aspirins and call the doctor in the morning

c. Call Emergency Medical Services (911) immediately

d. Have the victim drink caffeine, a stimulant

Notes

Notes

Part 3:
The Answers
and
Explanations

Notes

Answers and Explanations For The BLS Questions

1. How do you know if your ventilations are adequate, whether it is mouth to mask, bag mask ventilations, or mouth-to-mouth breaths?

c. The chest rises with each breath you administer. The best way to check for adequate breaths is to ensure there is an adequately open airway and then watch for chest rise while giving a slow deep breath.

2. What is the definition of the term "to recoil" completely after each chest compression?

c. Taking your weight off your hands and allow the chest to come back to its normal position. Recoil in CPR is when the chest is allowed to come back to a resting position after a chest compression. Compressions on all age groups are deep, fast, and hard, however allowing recoil assists with cardiac circulation.

3. In BLS, two minutes is considered 5 cycles. Within one cycle what is the ratio of compressions to ventilations in one-rescuer CPR (all ages)?

b. 30 compressions to 2 breaths. The ratio of compressions to ventilations in all age groups is 30 compressions to 2 breaths (30:2). The "rate" of compressions over a minute delivered is at least 100 compressions per minute. The only exceptions are: continuous chest compressions once a victim has an advanced airway inserted, or CPR for infants and child – two-rescuer CPR – 15 compressions to 2 breaths (15:2).

4. When a victim has fallen or there is trauma suspected, how does the rescuer open the victim's airway?

d. Use the modified jaw thrust maneuver. Always considering if a victim on the ground has a neck injury, a rescuer should attempt the modified jaw thrust method when opening the airway. This maneuver requires two hands to pull the jaw forward while blocking the victim's nose with your cheek while trying to ventilate, if using mouth to mouth. If necessary the rescuer may need to tilt the head back, as little as possible in order to get air into the victim. If there is no neck injury suspected, use the head tilt-chin lift maneuver.

5. How fast is the rate of compressions per minute for victims of any age?

b. At least 100 to 120 compressions per minute. The faster the compressions are the better the circulation, however it must be high quality compressions, with adequate recoil. With the ratio of 30 compressions to 2 breaths the average compression rate is at 100 to 120 compressions per minute.

6. What are the signs of adequate breathing from the victim? Looking at the chest is one of the signs. What other signs do you assess for?

c. Listening at the victim's mouth. Look for chest-rise for breathing, and listen at the victim's mouth for exhalation of air, to determine if the victim is breathing. If there is inadequate signs of breathing feel for a pulse, and if there is no pulse, then within 10 seconds begin chest compressions.

7. What is the best way for a rescuer to know that a rescue breath for an infant victim is effective?

c. The chest rises. Infants are considered "belly breathers", however it is chest rise and fall that lets us know air is getting into the lungs. If their belly and chest move together that is considered normal. If the movements are asynchronous – this is called rocking/paradoxical and it is not considered normal.

8. When a victim is barely breathing (agonal gasps), but has a pulse, and someone has called the emergency medical system (EMS), what should you do?

c. Open the airway, give 2 breaths, and then 1 breath every 5 to 6 seconds. It is safe to assist a victim with breaths when they are having difficulty breathing. Open the airway and attempt to give two breaths (as they inhale). If that works continue rescue breathing – one breath every 5 to 6 seconds, until the emergency team arrives (check the pulse if necessary). Use a barrier device (pocket mask, BMV) whenever possible.

9. When should a rescuer begin chest compressions with breaths (CPR) for an adult?

c. The adult is not responding, not breathing, and you cannot feel a pulse. Once the rescuer assesses that there is no breathing and you cannot feel a pulse, begin chest compressions with ventilations.

10. How is CPR done on infants ages birth to 1-year-old when there are two healthcare providers?

c. Cycles of 15 compressions and 2 breaths, with one rescuer giving chest compressions and the other giving the breaths. Only healthcare professionals learn about two-rescuer CPR. One rescuer does the compressions while the other rescuer gives the ventilations. The ratio for two-rescuer CPR is 15 compressions to 2 breaths.

11. How is CPR done on infants ages birth to 1-year-old when there is one healthcare provider?

a. One rescuer gives cycles of 30 compressions and 2 breaths. CPR is 30 compressions to 2 breaths for one rescuer, for all age groups. If there are two healthcare professionals performing CPR on infants, then 15 to 2 would be the ratio for compressions to ventilation.

12. What is the ratio and method for one-rescuer CPR on children ages 1 to 12-years-old?

a. Ratio is 30 compressions to 2 breaths using one or two hands. CPR ratio for one-rescuer child CPR is 30 compressions to 2 breaths. Compressions are done with the heel of one hand for small children (ages 1 to 8) and two hands for larger children (ages 8 to 12).

13. Why it is important to do fast and hard CPR and provide early defibrillation to an adult?

d. Successful defibrillation relies on the high quality CPR given continuously up to that time. High quality CPR with deep fast compressions, with good recoil, provides the heart muscle with the oxygen it needs to be successfully defibrillated. If high quality CPR is done for 2 to 4 minutes the defibrillation (unsynchronized cardioversion) is up to 90% successful.

14. What is the first thing to be done when the automatic external defibrillator (AED) is brought to the side of a cardiac arrest victim?

b. Turn on the AED, apply pads to the victim's chest. Turning the AED on assists the rescuer because it will audibly tell you what the steps are to operate the AED and when to continue CPR. It recognizes errors as well, such as pad placement and if the plug for the pads is not secured properly.

15. At what time during the cardiac arrest rescue are the automatic external defibrillator (AED) pads applied?

d. The AED pads are applied as soon as they are made available. While the first rescuer is performing CPR, a second rescuer will bring over the AED and turn it on. The AED will immediately direct the second rescuer to "apply pads to the victim's bare chest. Plug in connector, STAND CLEAR, analyzing rhythm, and to press the shock button" if necessary.

16. What could happen if you or someone in the team or crowd is touching the victim while the AED is delivering a shock?

c. The AED could shock you while it is shocking the victim. If anyone is touching the victim or even the equipment/bed, there is a risk of the shock reaching the one in contact. In the hospital the respiratory therapists have been at the highest risk. For these reasons it is very important to say "ALL CLEAR" prior to pressing the shock button.

17. When using an AED, and the AED says "no shock advised", what should you do next?

d. Leave the pads on the victim's chest and continue with compressions. You must return to CPR. When the AED analyzes and the message is "no shock advised", the patient does not have a shockable rhythm. The victim is not in a shockable rhythm such as ventricular fibrillation or pulseless ventricular tachycardia. The victim most likely still requires the continuation of CPR. Leave the pads on so the AED can reanalyze.

18. An adult victim standing next to you has an obstructed airway, how will you help this choking victim?

b. Perform abdominal thrusts until the obstruction is relieved or victim is unconscious. Inward and upward abdominal thrusts (at waist level) are very effective in relieving obstructions in a conscious victim. If the victim is unconscious begin chest compressions.

19. The abdominal thrusts are not working to relieve an obstructed airway. The victim becomes unconscious and you slide him/her onto their back. The waiter has already called 911. What should you do next?

c. Begin chest compressions immediately, always looking for the object to come out. To relieve the obstruction in the unconscious adult you begin chest compressions and ventilations (30:2). Chest compressions increase intra-thoracic pressure and assist with relieving the obstruction.

20. You begin the steps of CPR on an infant you find who is not responding at a daycare center. When should you call the emergency medical system (EMS)?

d. Call (or have someone call) EMS as soon as you find the unconscious infant. If the victim is unresponsive, advanced measures will be needed. This is why it is recommended to call 911 (EMS) as soon as possible in any emergency. If the victim is conscious with an obstructed airway, it is worth trying a simple maneuver to relieve the obstruction. Any other emergency situation - call 911 immediately. You must begin your ABC's (airway, breathing, circulation), now CAB's, as soon as possible.

21. There are two health professionals performing BLS on an infant. What is the correct ratio for chest compressions and ventilations for two-rescuer child CPR?

a. 15 compressions to 2 breaths. The child CPR ratio, when there are two rescuers is 15 compressions to 2 breaths (15:2). This assists with faster ventilation rates.

22. How do you relieve choking in conscious children and adults?

b. Perform abdominal thrusts until the object comes out, or the victim becomes unconscious. To rescue a conscious choking child between the ages of 1 and 12 years, or adult, the rescuer will stand behind the victim, and place his own thumb knuckle into the victim's umbilicus (waist line). The other hand will come around to the front of the child from the other side, and grab the fist and pull the abdomen inward and upward. Continue inward and upward thrusts until the object comes out or the victim becomes unconscious. If victim becomes unconscious, begin CPR.

23. Why are chest compressions done fast, hard, and with minimal interruptions to victims of any age?

b. Minimizing interruptions leads to improved blood flow and a higher rate of survival. Chest compressions are done fast and hard, with minimal interruptions, to increase adequate blood flow to the heart muscle. This increases the success of defibrillation and outcomes of cardiac arrest victims.

24. A pulseless child is receiving CPR, and an AED is brought to the scene. There aren't any pediatric pads available. Pediatric pads have an attenuator, that dramatically reduce the joules delivered. At this time can you use adult pads on the child?

a. Yes, but make sure the pads do not touch each other. If CPR has been initiated on a 1 to 12-year-old child, an AED is brought over and there are only adult pads available, then you CAN use them! Use both pads, but make sure they are not touching each other. The front and back of the chest method of placement may be safer if it is possible to get to the child's backs. The maximum joules for children is 10 J/kg or 200 joules maximum.

25. When the paramedic team arrives, they successfully insert an endotracheal tube into the victim's airway. The recommended rate for ventilations through the advanced airway is slower. What is the ventilatory rate for this victim?

d. One breath every 6 to 8 seconds. Once the victim has a properly placed advanced airway and is receiving 100% oxygen, slow down the rate to one breath every 6 to 8 seconds which amounts to 8 to 10 breaths/min in all age groups.

26. You are holding the choking infant in your arms. What is the most effective way to remove the obstructed object in the still conscious/awake infant?

b. Cycles of 5 backslaps, and 5 chest compressions, until the infant becomes unconscious, then begin CPR. Hold the infant on your arm, preferably leaning on your leg with the infants head faced down, straddling the legs on you upper arm. Perform cycles of 5 back slaps between the infants shoulder blades and turn the baby over onto the other arm and perform 5 chest compressions with 2 fingers (1-1/2 inches deep) one fingerbreadth below the nipple line, mid-sternum, repeating until the object comes out or the infant becomes unconscious. Begin CPR if the infant becomes unconscious.

27. How often should the rescuers switch during 2-rescuer adult CPR?

d. Every 5 cycles of 30 compressions to 2 breaths. Chest compressions are at 2 to 2-1/2 inches deep in the adult at the rate of at 100 to 120 compressions per minute. This fast and hard CPR is not easy and can tire a rescuer. Switching with another rescuer can continue high quality CPR for longer period of times. If compressors are not pressing hard enough, tell them to press harder. Coaching is an important part of teamwork.

28. CPR should be started prior to the AED application and initiated immediately after . . . ?

c. The defibrillation is delivered. It has been proven that the chest compressions within 10 seconds prior to and directly after a defibrillation increases the perfusion of blood in the body and successful return of spontaneous circulation (ROSC) by 53 %.

29. When compressing the infant's chest the rescuer must compress the chest how many inches?

a. 1-1/2 inches. Chest compressions on infant victims is at least 1/3 the depth of the chest or 1-1/2 inches deep. Infants are less than 1-year-of-age.

30. How long should a rescuer take when checking a victim's responsiveness, breathing and pulse?

a. The rescuer should check for response, breathing, and for a pulse, within 10 seconds. Once finding an unresponsive victim, you must call emergency services. If the victim is not responding, begin hard and fast chest compressions.

31. The AED can be obtained and turned on by . . . ?

d. All of the above. Anyone, regardless of their training, can operate an automatic external defibrillator. When you turn it on it tells you what to do. There are also pictures provided to show you what to do. So, always turn the AED on, as soon as possible. Certainly it is better to have some training in the AED, and there are many manufacturers that make different models.

32. The automatic external defirillator (AED) can save a life by . . . ?

d. All of the above. Recognizing pulseless ventricular rhythms, advising rescuers to continue chest compressions, and advising the rescuers a defibrillation is needed. The AED recognizes shockable rhythms, tells you when to press the shock button, and advises the rescuer to continue chest compressions.

33. Practicing and testing with the AED and pads is mandatory in CPR/BLS courses because . . . ?

d. Both b and c. Practicing pad placement will prepare you for the real situation. And, coordinated team efforts with the AED and compressions lead to greater success. Chest compressions should not be stopped while the pads are placed on the victim's chest. This team effort will lead to greater success stories.

34. The best place to check a pulse on an infant is . . . ?

c. The brachial artery. The brachial artery is the best place to access an arterial pulse on the infant. It is easy to access and palpate on the infant.

35. The best place to check a pulse on a child is . . . ?

a. The carotid artery. This is the easiest and strongest pulse to access in children and adults. It is fairly easy to locate on either side of the neck. In the hospital the femoral artery is palpated for the patient because the patient has clothes on.

36. The best place to check a pulse on an adult is . . . ?
a. The carotid artery. The carotid artery is the easiest and strongest pulse to access in children and adults. It is fairly easy to locate on either side of the neck. The femoral artery is often palpated on unconscious patients in the hospital.

37. The child is considered to be between the ages of 1-year and 12-years-of-age. Ages 1 through 8 are considered "small" children. What is the technique for chest compressions for the small child?
b. The heel of one hand. The heel of one hand is used to compress the child's chest 2 inches deep. If the child is over eight years old and is large – 2 hands are used.

38. How are chest compressions (2 inches deep) performed on a large child ages 8 to 12?
a. Two hands. One or two-hand is used for child CPR. For large children, two hands will assist in consistent 2-inch depth of compressions.

39. When opening the airway of an unconscious infant victim, the technique used is often called . . . ?
a. The sniffing position. The sniffing position is just a slight lift of the head - pointing the nose toward the ceiling - mimicking a sniff - to open the airway.

40. When assessing the victim for responsiveness, you should . . . ?
d. All of the above. Watch for his chest rise and fall, and listen for exhaled air by the victim's mouth and nose. Also, check the pulse for 10 seconds. If the patient appears unresponsive call emergency medical services.

41. If the infant/child is unresponsive and you are alone, you should . . . ?

c. Begin the CAB of CPR and activate the emergency medical services immediately. If you are alone with an unconscious victim you should activate the emergency medical service as soon as possible. Beginning the CAB/ABC's of CPR. Begin chest compressions if needed.

42. When ventilating a child with a bag mask device . . . ?

b. Ventilate to see rise and fall of the chest. Rise and fall of the chest indicates enough air in the chest. A larger breath can cause gastric distention, vomiting and aspiration pneumonia.

43. Chest compressions on an infant is performed at what depth?

c. 1-1/2 inches deep, one finger breath below the nipple line. The proper depth of compression for infant CPR is 1-1/2-inch deep. This is at least 1/3 the chest anterior / posterior diameter, just below the nipple line using two fingers, or two thumbs.

44. Which is the most effective method of chest compressions in two-rescuer CPR for the infant victim?

d. The two-thumb technique. The two-thumb technique - with the hands wrapped around the infant's back squeezing the sternum 1-1/2 inches deep offers a better cardiac output in 2-rescuer CPR.

45. Chest compressions on a child is performed at what depth?

d. 2 inches deep. Two inches or 5 cms is the proper depth at the rate of at 100 to 120 compressions per minute, for the child victim.

46. Chest compressions on an adult is performed at what depth?

d. 2 to 2-1/2 inches deep. At the rate of 100 to 120 compressions per minute for the adult victim.

47. When performing the abdominal thrusts on a conscious choking child or adult, how do you know you are doing it successfully?

d. Both b and c. The choking victim begins to cough and breath on their own, and pulling your fist inward and upward from the victims waistline. Pulling your fist inward and upward from the victims waistline. This will hopefully relieve the obstruction. The choking victim begins to cough and breath on their own. This victim has been relieved of their obstruction.

48. When the conscious choking victim becomes unconscious and is gently placed on the ground the rescuer must . . . ?

a. Call the emergency medical services and begin chest compressions and ventilations (30:2). The best method to relieve an obstruction in the unconscious victim is chest compressions. Once the obstruction is relieved the rescuer can remove the object, ventilate, and if the victim is resuscitated – placed in the recovery (side) position awaiting emergency services.

49. When doing chest compressions at the victim's side and you are alone, which ventilation device or method would be the most difficult to perform alone and take the most time to use?

c. Bag-mask ventilation. The bag mask device is perfect for a second rescuer who is at the victim's head and can hold the mask and squeeze bag when appropriate, between compressions.

50. Before approaching a victim in an unfamiliar environment the rescuer must . . . ?

d. Both a and b. Call the emergency medical services, and ensure that area is safe to approach. Before approaching a situation it is important that you are safe. Perfect examples are a drowning scene. You must be able to throw a lifesaver rope or ring, or hold on to the pool ladder rather than being pulled under by a frantic drowning victim. Call 911 immediately in any emergency situation.

51. If the AED is not working properly, what should be done immediately?

c. Immediately start chest compressions. It would take too much time to try to repair the AED, continue high-quality chest compressions for the most favorable outcome.

52. The Basic Life Support (BLS) Certification card needs renewal every . . . ?

c. 2 years. Many institutions require renewal of BLS certification at minimum every two years. Some may require an annual training.

53. An infant appears to be choking, what are the signs and symptoms of an infant choking?

c. The infant will make high pitch sounds and may turn bluish. There will be signs of hypoxia: circumoral (mouth) and periorbital (eyes) cyanosis (bluish color).

54. What is the procedure to relieve an obstruction in the conscious choking infant?

d. Perform 5 back slaps and 5 chest compressions. If the victim becomes unconscious, begin CPR.

55. What are the signs and symptoms of a child choking?

c. The child can make high pitch sounds or be silent. The small area by the vocal cords is the part of the anatomy where objects can get lodged.

56. What is the procedure to relieve an obstructed airway in a conscious choking child?

a. Perform abdominal thrusts. Perform inward and upward abdominal thrusts at the waist-line/umbilical area, until the object is dislodged. If the child becomes unconscious, begin CPR.

57. An adult appears to be choking, what are the signs and symptoms of an adult choking?

a. The adult will be silent, and may raise their arms to their neck. Raising the arms to the neck is called the "Universal Sign of Choking". Choking adults often walk or run away due to embarrassment of coughing and choking. If you recognize these signs, follow the victim and call for help.

58. What is the procedure to relieve an obstructed airway in a conscious choking adult?

a. Perform abdominal thrusts. Perform abdominal thrusts by pulling in ward and upward with your fist at the level of the umbilicus/waistline, until the obstruction is relieved, or the victim becomes unconscious. Lie the victim on the ground and begin CPR.

59. If a choking victim of any age becomes unconscious, what should the rescuer do?

b. Call 911 (EMS) and begin chest compressions. CPR may assist in dislodging the obstruction, but the emergency services will be on the way if advanced airway support is needed.

60. You have cleared the airway on an unconscious choking victim, doing high-quality chest compressions. You already called 911 (EMS). What should you do now?

a. Check for breathing and pulse. Continue CPR if needed, or turn the victim on their side.

61. You have cleared the airway on an unconscious choking victim. There is a pulse and the victim is breathing. What should you do now?

a. Turn the victim on the side - the recovery/rescue position. This will prevent any aspiration and assists the victim in breathing on their own.

62. What equipment would a rescuer need to perform Basic Life Support?

b. A pocket mask/face shield and an AED. This is the basic equipment to enhance a rescue. The pocket mask would enable the health care provider to safely deliver breaths until other equipment arrives at the scene. Once you begin CPR, the victim's best chance for survival would be if an automatic external defibrillator was applied and it analyzed and defibrillated the victim.

63. The AED is an . . . ?

b. Automatic External Defibrillator. The automatic external defibrillator will analyze a shockable rhythm and deliver approximately 200 to 360 joules when used properly. Each AED manufacturer may have a different amount of joules delivered.

64. The AED is equipped with defibrillator pads. What sizes are usually available in the hospital setting?

d. Adult, child, and infant size pads are available. The pads are made by different manufacturers. The infant and child size pads are often combination pads.

65. What if you only have pediatric pads available? Can you use them on an adult?

a. No, the energy is not high enough, begin chest compressions. The pediatric pads deliver approximately 50 joules. That is not enough energy to successfully defibrillate an adult victim.

66. Are all AED pad connectors universal and fit into every AED or defibrillator cable?

b. No, pads and connectors are not universal. Every AED and defibrillator may require its own manufactured pad. The pads also have expiration dates.

67. What is the compression depth for an infant of 8-months-old?

c. 1-1/2 inches deep. Adult compression depth is 2 to 2-1/2 inches, and children compressions are 2 inches deep.

68. Two health professionals are doing CPR on an infant. One rescuer is ventilating, and the other is compressing. Which technique is used for two-rescuer CPR for the infant victim?

a. The two-thumb compression technique, with the fingers around the infants back. This is the preferred technique for two rescuers. One rescuer is doing the compressions and the other will be providing the ventilations.

69. What is the depth of chest compressions for a child, ages 1 to 12-years-old?

d. 2 inches deep. This is the depth of compressions for children, at the rate of 100 to 120 compressions per minute.

70. What is the depth of chest compressions on an adult victim with no pulse?

d. 2 to 2-1/2 inches deep. Allow full recoil, and compress at the rate of at least 100 compressions per minute, for 2 minutes or 5 cycles of 30 compressions to 2 breaths.

71. What is the ratio of compressions to ventilations for one or two-rescuer adult CPR?

a. 30 compressions : 2 breaths (30:2).

72. What is the ratio of compressions to ventilations for one-rescuer infant or child CPR?

c. 30 compressions : 2 breaths (30:2). The ration to compressions in one rescuer CPR for all age groups is 30 compressions : 2 breaths (30:2). Two-rescuer CPR for infants and children is 15 compressions to 2 breaths (15:2).

73. What is the ratio of compressions to ventilations for two-rescuer infant or child CPR?

c. 15 compressions : 2 breaths (15:2).

74. What is the placement position of the two AED pads for an effective defibrillation?

c. Left side at the lower rib cage, and below the right clavicle. An alternative placement is in the front and back of the chest, but may not be the quickest way to place pads during a cardiac arrest situation.

75. If the infant victim requires airway support and ventilation using the bag-mask, how will you know if the breaths are adequate?

d. There will be rise and fall of the chest with adequate breaths. Squeeze the bag about half of its size, enough to get adequate rise and fall of the chest for adequate breaths.

76. What is the proper ventilation rate for infant and child rescue-breathing?

d. One breath every 3 to 5 seconds. One breath every 3 to 5 seconds is the proper rate of ventilations for infants and children. If there is an advanced airway (with 100% oxygen), slow the breaths down to one breath every 6 to 8 seconds.

77. When compressing the chest of an adult, where is the correct placement of your hands?

b. Two hands on the lower one-half of the sternum/breastbone. Correct placement for adult CPR is two hands on the lower one half of the sternum/breastbone, pressing down 2 to 2-1/2 inches, and relaxing hand in between compressions allowing for complete chest recoil.

78. Mechanical devices that assist and improve CPR delivery are . . . ?

d. All of the above. Chest compression measurement and feedback device, the automatic chest compression (thumper) machine, and the capnograph device (measurement of exhaled CO2), all can be used by healthcare professionals to improve the outcomes of cardiac arrest.

79. When a victim has an occluded airway, what part of the anatomy is obstructed?

c. The vocal cords and trachea. The area where we choke is the small area in the upper airway.

80. The abdominal thrust are not working to relieve the obstructed airway in the victim. Just prior to the victim becoming unconscious, what other lifesaving maneuvers might work?

d. Both a and b. Chest thrust, from behind the choking victim, and back slaps. Abdominal thrust is the most effective. Chest thrust, from behind the choking victim and back slaps is another alternative to the abdominal thrusts, especially for pregnant or obese victims. However, if the victim becomes unconscious, lower them gently to the ground, call 911, and begin chest compression.

81. If you are alone and an adult needs resuscitation what should you do first?

d. Phone emergency medical services (911). Do this as soon as possible. You may be able to use a cellphone and begin CPR simultaneously.

82. A choking child becomes unconscious and is on the floor. What should you do?

d. Phone emergency services (911). And then begin chest compressions.

83. What is the survival rate for CPR?

a. The adult survival rate from out-of-hospital cardiac arrest is about 2 to 15%.

84. What will increase the survival rate for cardiac arrest victims?

b. Using the automatic external defibrillator (AED). Using the automatic external defibrillator (AED) after 2 minutes of high quality CPR may increase the survival rate in victims of cardiac arrest.

85. Why is debriefing important after a team intervention occurs?

c. Review the event afterwards to see what went well and what could have gone better.

86. Who is required to take the BLS program for healthcare providers?

b. Paramedics, physicians, and nurses. Advanced airway techniques are taught in the healthcare provider course. CPR for all ages is also included in this program.

87. A 78-year-old woman tells you, "I think I am having a stroke". What are the signs and symptoms you are looking for?

d. All of the above. Weakness and numbness on one side of her body, slurred speech, and facial droop. Weakness and numbness and "arm drift" on one side of the body is common. Slurred speech is detected by asking the victim to repeat a short phrase. Facial droop on one side is a sign you are looking for when the victim tries to smile.

88. What is universal precautions, and what is needed to perform CPR?

c. Universal precautions protect from infectious diseases, and you need gloves and a pocket mask. A bag-mask-valve device can also be used.

89. You are doing compressions on an adult victim. The automatic external defibrillator (AED) only has pediatric pads. What are you doing next?

b. Continue chest compressions. Pediatric joule dosing (50 J) is not adequate for an adult.

90. You are caring for a 6-month-old infant, whose condition has been deteriorating. When would you begin chest compressions on an infant?

a. Begin chest compressions on the infant if the heart rate is less than 60 beats per minute. A heart rate less than 60 in infants and children, despite treatments, represents a hypoxic and dying heart, so you must start CPR.

91. How often should you check a pulse on adults, infants and children, once CPR has been initiated?

c. A pulse should be checked with every two-minute CPR switch. Switching every two minutes gives the team time to switch compressors, identify if a defibrillation is required, as well as checking the pulse.

92. What is the typical cause of cardiac arrest in children?

b. Progressive deterioration in respiratory function is the typical cause of cardiac arrest.

93. Why is the two-thumb technique more effective for infant CPR?

c. The two-thumb technique produces better blood flow, and consistent depth and artificial blood pressure (perfusion).

94. What are the implications of a victim lying on wet ground, when applying the automatic external defibrillator (AED)?

d. Both a and b. The victim can be lying in wet area if it is impossible to move the victim, and the victim's chest should be as dry as possible. The victim should be moved from the wet area if possible. However, if the victim cannot be moved, be sure all bystanders are away from the victim. The chest should be as dry as possible or the shock will go across the water on the chest – not into the chest. The chest should be dried to allow the pads to stick to the skin.

95. Why is it important to avoid applying the automatic external defibrillator (AED) pads on top of medicated patches?

d. The medicated patch can actually cause burns on the skin and prevent the joules being delivered to the victim.

96. The victim is pulseless and breathless. Emergency services are on their way. You begin chest compressions. Another rescuer asks if they can help. What will you tell the second rescuer to do?

d. Both a and c. The second rescuer should get the nearest AED and apply the pads. Then the second rescuer should begin the ventilations. Ratio of 30 compressions to 2 breaths (30:2) for the adult. And 15:2 for infants and children, 2-rescuer CPR. The EMS was notified already.

97. The Good Samaritan Law are laws or acts offering legal protection to people who give reasonable assistance to those who are injured, ill, in peril, or otherwise incapacitated outside the hospital setting. This law applies to . . . ?

d. All of the above. Physician and Nurses; therapist or registered physician's assistant; and the general public. The only time a law suit can be pursued is if it established that such injuries were, or such death was caused by, gross negligence on the part of such person.

98. A myocardial infarction (heart attack) may ultimately lead to cardiac arrest depending on the severity of the blockage in the heart. What are the signs and symptoms of a heart attack?

d. Both a and b. Chest pain, and nausea, vomiting and diaphoresis (sweating). Other symptoms may include jaw pain, left arm pain, back pain, and shortness of breath. Blurred vision is not a typical symptom.

99. When a victim has chest pain and you already have called the Emergency Medical Services (911), what else can you do while waiting for the ambulance?

b. See if the victim can chew a regular aspirin. The paramedics will have the victim chew a regular aspirin (160 mg to 325 mg).

100. Stroke is a disease of physical complications including weakness and paralysis. What are the signs and symptoms of stroke?

d. All of the above. Slurred speech, headache and sensory loss, and vision changes. Symptoms can be minor or severe. Always call 911. Getting to the emergency department in a timely fashion is extremely important. An initial non-contrast CAT Scan is done within 25 minutes of arrival and tPA is administered in the first 3 to 4-1/2 hours of the onset of symptoms, if it is a clot or ischemic stroke.

101. When a victim has the signs and symptoms of stroke what is the best immediate action to take?

c. Call Emergency Medical Services (911) immediately. The paramedics will know how to assess and treat the stroke patient. It is actually dangerous to give the victim liquids to drink, for their ability to swallow is often effected. The victim can choke and aspirate.

Notes

Notes

Part 4:
The Appendix

Notes

Glossary

Abdomen: a cavity that holds the stomach, intestines, liver, kidneys, pancreas and spleen.

Abdominal thrust (Heimlich Maneuver): a rescuer standing behind a choking victim using their fists at waist-line (umbilicus)to pull the abdomen inward and upwards until the obstruction is pushed up and out of the diaphragm.

Abrasion: superficial damage to skin, no deeper than the epidermis.

Accident: focus on physical trauma that can result in injury, disability and death. Mostly from motor vehicle accidents, falls, penetrating wounds, burns, violence, and drug abuse.

Activate EMS / 911: once recognizing that an emergency situation exists, it is the first action in the "chain of survival" (early access, early CPR, early defibrillation, and early advanced cardiac life support).

Airway support: includes the head-tilt chin lift, jaw-thrust maneuvers, and infant "sniffing position", when encouraging breathing, initiating oxygen therapy, or bag-mask-ventilation.

Advanced airway support: oral or nasopharyngeal airways, criothyrotomy, intubation using laryngoscopes or LMA (laryngeal mask airways. Oral or nasal endotracheal tubes or surgical procedures to insert tracheostomy tubes.

AED (automatic external defibrillator): semi-automatic, portable device that recognizes pulseless ventricular dysrhythmias and can deliver a defibrillation (shock).

Agonal gasps: refers to the last breaths taken prior to death. Agonal rhythm: refers to the last heart beats seen on a cardiac monitor prior to death.

Airway: throat, larynx, trachea.

AMBU bag: Artificial Manual Breathing Unit: used to provide positive pressure ventilation to a victim/patient who is not breathing adequately.

Angina: chest pain due to ischemia (lack of blood) to the heart muscle, caused by obstruction or spasm of the coronary arteries.

Arrhythmia: disruption of the normal electrical cycle and cardiac rhythm. Can be life threatening.

Artery: blood vessels that carry oxygenated blood from the heart to the body parts.

Asynchronous: not simultaneous.

Asystole: no cardiac activity or contractions.

Atropine (belladonna): an anticholinergic drug that increases heart rates, dilates pupils, and reduces secretions.

Back slaps: used to dislodge obstructions in unconscious choking infants, with the heel of one hand in-between the infant's shoulder blades.

Belly breathers: diaphragmatic breathing where the stomach moves as seen with infants.

BLS / BCLS: Basic Life Support: (older term is Basic Cardiac Life Support) is medical support for airway and circulation emergencies; includes CPR.

Brachial artery: palpated in the upper inner aspect of the upper arm. Common area to feel for an infant's pulse.

Bradycardia: resting heart rate under 60 beats per minute (bpm).

CABs (formerly ABCs): Circulation-Airway-Breathing: the priorities in BLS.

Cardiac arrest: see: Sudden cardiac arrest.

Cardiovascular: blood vessel and heart components of the circulatory system.

Carotid Artery: palpated on either side of the Adam's apple.

Child: (small) ages 1 -8, (large) ages 8-12 (for BLS guidelines).

Circumoral cyanosis: bluish coloring around mouth from hypoxia.

Compression-to-ventilation ratio: number of chest compressions to ventilations. Eg: adults CPR is 30:2.

Contusion: a closed wound, bruise.

Coronary arteries: the initial vessels off the aorta feeding the heart muscle.

CPR (cardio-pulmonary-resuscitation): chest compressions and ventilations.

Cyanosis (bluish color): blue or purple coloration of skin or mucus membranes due to hypoxia (lack of oxygen).

Defibrillation (cardioversion): delivery of electrical energy (joules) to correct a life-threatening dysrhythmia.

Diaphragm: thin muscle in chest cavity contracts to draw air into the lungs.

DNR: (Do Not Resuscitate/no code): a legal order and/or patient request to allow a natural death.

ECG: (ECG-electrocardiogram): recording of the electrical activity of the heart.

EMS: emergency medical services: providing out-of-hospital acute medical care, and transport to the appropriate facility.

EMT / Paramedic: pre-hospital providers of basic life support that have advanced training.

Femoral artery: a site for palpating a pulse is in the upper inner thigh, at the groin. Presence of a femoral pulse indicates a systolic blood pressure of more than 50 mmHg.

Finger sweep: method of removal of a foreign body from the mouth when visualized.

First-aid: initial care for an illness or injury. Eg; burns, bites, stings, rashes, scrapes, splinters and cuts.

First responder: person who arrives first at the scene of an incident. May be dispatched by the ambulance service, may be passers-by, citizen volunteers, or may be the police or fire department.

Good Samaritan Law: legal protection intended to reduce bystanders' hesitation to assist, for fear of being sued or prosecuted for unintentional injury or wrongful death.

Gurney: stretcher.

Head-tilt chin-lift: opening the airway; one hand lifts the chin and the other tilts the head back by the forehead.

Heart attack (myocardial infarction): spasm or clogging of a coronary artery due to coronary artery disease.

Heel-of-one-hand technique: chest compressions on small children is done with the heel of one hand.

High quality CPR: performing chest compressions fast and hard with recoil.

Hyperventilate: breathing too fast.

Hypotension: low blood pressure which is causing symptoms.

Hypothermia: low body temperature. Below 36.5°C (98 °F).

Hypoxia: lack of oxygen in blood and tissue.

Infant: a baby between the ages of 1 month and 1 year.

Infarction: (necrosis) tissue death.

Intra-thoracic pressure: pressure within the chest cavity.

Intubation: insertion of an advanced airway or tube.

Ischemia: restriction of blood supply to tissues/organs.

Jaw-thrust maneuver: method to open the airway on patients with a suspected spinal injury. The rescuers use their own thumbs to physically push the jaw forward.

Joules: the amount of electrical energy from the AED, or defibrillator; e.g. 200 J.

Laceration: skin is torn, cut or punctured.

Lay person: non-professional.

Mouth-to-mouth ventilations: delivering breaths by mouth if there are no alternative devices.

Neonate: newborn from birth to 1 month old.

Obstruction (airway): an object blocking the trachea.

Pacemaker: medical device that uses electrical impulses (mAs: milliamperes) to regulate the heart's beating.

Palpation: feeling/examining the patient with your hands.

Palpitation: abnormal heartbeat which can be a symptom of an illnesses.

Paramedic: provider of out-of-hospital treatment and some diagnostic services, and medical treatment of minor injuries. Highest licensure level of pre-hospital emergency care.

Pericardium: membrane which covers the heart; protects and lubricates the heart.

Periorbital cyanosis: bluish color around the eyes from hypoxia.

Pocket mask/face mask/face shield: a device used to safely deliver mouth to mouth breaths during a cardiac arrest or respiratory arrest.

Pulmonary: refers to the lungs and respiration system.

Recoil: with each deep chest compressions; returning to the chest's normal position.

Respiration: the exchange of oxygen and carbon dioxide between the atmosphere and the body cells; diffusion of oxygen from alveoli to blood and of carbon dioxide from blood to alveoli; and transport of oxygen to and carbon dioxide from body cells.

Resuscitate: to restore consciousness or life to.

Shock: circulatory or hypovolemic shock: the organs and tissues are not receiving an adequate flow of blood.

Shock: mental shock: a psychological condition in response to a terrifying or traumatic event, with feelings of intense helplessness.

Shockable rhythm: ventricular fibrillation and ventricular tachycardia with no palpable pulses.

Sniffing position: the optimal position for an infants airway. A slight tilt of the head - backward, pointing the nose upward.

Splints: device used for support or immobilization of limbs and the spine.

Sprain: joint injury caused by ligament being stretched beyond capacity.

Sternum: breastbone; press on the lower one-half of the sternum for chest compressions.

Subcutaneous tissue: Hypodermis: lowermost layer of skin.

Sudden cardiac arrest / cardiac arrest: the cessation of normal circulation of the blood due to failure of the heart to contract effectively. The heart is fibrillating or not beating at all.

Symptoms: any evidence of disease or a patient's condition, i.e., such evidence as perceived by the patient; a change in a patient's condition indicative of some bodily or mental state.

Tachycardia: resting heart rate over 100 beats per min (bpm).

Telemetry: electronically monitoring, measuring, and recording patient medical data and vital signs for analysis.

Tertiary facility: a facility or hospital that can provide special services and medical surgical care to the critically ill or injured.

Trauma: serious and body-altering physical injury, such as the removal of a limb.

Triage: the process of determining the priority of patients' treatments based on the severity of their condition.

Two-thumb technique: a two-rescuer technique for infant CPR, where one rescuer places two hands around the infants chest and back. The fingers are wrapped under the arms and the two-thumbs are pressing on the sternum.

Umbilicus: refers to the navel/belly button at the waist line.

Ventilation: including inhalation and exhalation.

About the Authors

Michele G. Kunz, MSN, ANP, RN-BC

Michele is an AHA Certified Instructor and specializes in providing AHA Certification classes in ACLS, BLS, and PALS. Visit her website to see more about her classes, books, study guides, essays, and articles. Visit Michele's YouTube page to see all of her free video lessons.

Michele has been a clinical nursing educator for over 32 years. During those years, she has helped many thousands of nurses improve their own job performance and increase their own job satisfaction. Michele considers herself to be a nurse's nurse, because she is not hidden away in a classroom or office, but out on the floor everyday – interacting with hospital management, the nurses, the patients, and the physicians.

For many years Kunz was the Director of Nursing Education and Informatics at Long Island College Hospital in Brooklyn, NY. She was in the LICH Nursing Education Department for 25 years. Kunz developed the desire to teach nurses over 30 years ago when she was an ICU nurse at Staten Island University Hospital. It was at SIUH that Kunz realized that she could learn how to be a better nurse by teaching the other nurses. Kunz hasn't stopped teaching since then.

Kunz is now teaching in the Department of Nursing Education at Mercy Medical Center in Rockville Centre, Long Island, NY.

She is also the Director of Education at Dickson Keanaghan, LLC, a company that she helped create, where Michele and Joe train and certify the medical staff of over 600 hospitals, medical offices, and surgi-centers on Long Island and New York City. If you would like to take one of her classes, or have her come to your office and train your staff, please visit her training website at MicheleKunz.com. Connect with Michele on LinkedIn at http://www. linkedin.com/in/nursingeducatormichelegkunz

Joseph C. Kunz, Jr., MBA, BA

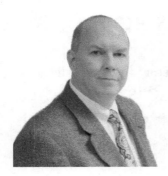

When Joe and Michele met in 1984, Michele was working full-time in the Intensive Care Unit at Staten Island University Hospital, and teaching a few classes on the side. Joe was building his first start-up company on Long Island, and began assisting Michele with the classes. By 1985 they realized that they wanted to take their little part-time training business to the next level. So, the two of them took a part-time weekend job at a nursing service in Brooklyn where they taught certification classes to nurses and physicians. Michele taught the classes, and Joe learned all about managing the business, the classes, the students, the classroom, the other instructors, and the equipment.

Eventually the Kunz's started to teach more classes on their own. They very quickly built a dedicated following of nurses and physicians throughout New York City and Long Island. They then started to grow the company very quickly and began training and certifying the medical staff at medical offices and then entire hospitals.

The Kunz's business would not be as successful as it is without the both of them working together. Right from the beginning Joe brought all his business experience and entrepreneurial fortitude into the operation. Joe had been developing his business skills and work-ethic from a very young age. He has worked very hard at making the business professional, successful, and strong. Over these last 32 years, Michele has perfected the teaching part of our operation, and Joe has perfected the marketing, management, and financial side.

The Kunz's business has been a wonderful 32+ year learning experience and journey. Despite the long days and hard work, they never want their journey to end. Each are looking forward to seeing how far they can take it. The more healthcare professionals and students that they help, the more successful they both feel. Joseph is a Certified Instructor for BLS. Connect with Joe on LinkedIn at www.linkedin.com/in/josephckunzjr/

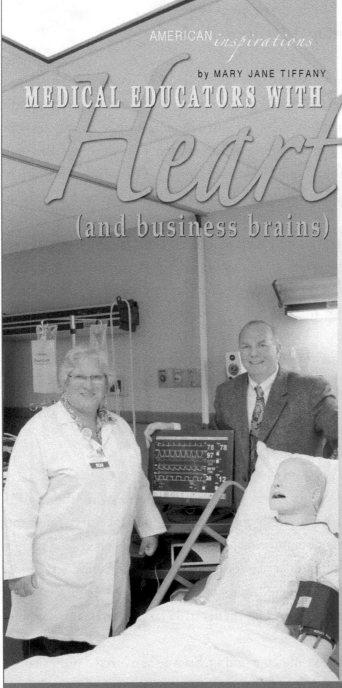

AMERICAN *inspirations*

by MARY JANE TIFFANY

MEDICAL EDUCATORS WITH
Heart
(and business brains)

Michele and Joe Kunz have created a business based on their love of teaching, helping others be successful, and for being together. Michele proudly says "teaching and sharing information is our life's mission."

Together they have been on the front-line of teaching and certifying healthcare professionals and students since 1984. They saw that there was a great need for educators that loved their subject matter, and that would treat their students with the respect they deserved. They have since built their medical training company into one of New York City's and Long Island's most popular American Heart Association certification companies. They train and certify the medical staff at over 600 hospitals, surgi-centers, medical offices, and universities.

Michele has been in nursing education for over 30 years. She is also the Director of Nursing Education at Mercy Medical Center on Long Island. Joe has been a business innovator and entrepreneur for over 30 years. He has been building and managing their business and finding and creating new and better ways to reach out and help more healthcare professionals be successful.

Over the years their classroom study materials developed a large national following. "In the early days we were creating, using, and distributing our own study materials before any existed in the marketplace," Joe recalls. "Healthcare professionals and students were desperate for easy-to-use study materials. So we created them." In 2003 they finally decided to branch into publishing with their *Zombie Notes*® study charts and books. They have been national best-sellers for the last several years.

The Kunzs have built their careers on providing fun, practical, timely, and informative classes, study materials, and videos that assist healthcare professionals and students in making our world a better place to live. Clearly, the art of educating is their passion, and it is one that Michele and Joe Kunz cherish. ▣

TheNurseEducator.com
MicheleKunz.com

Mary Jane Tiffany is a business professor at a major university in Texas and the author of several entrepreneurship books. She writes extensively on entrepreneurial couples.

About Dickson Keanaghan

Our Medical Training Adventure Begins

We developed the *Zombie Notes Study Charts* in 1984, when we first started teaching certification classes in New York City. Back then, there were no practical or effective study guides for our students to use or buy. So we had to develop our own study material to help prepare our students for the class. We very quickly learned what works with our students and what doesn't. Our classes and study guides very quickly developed a very large local audience in Manhattan and Brooklyn.

The nurses and physicians in our classes would then call us to come to their offices and hospitals to train and certify their entire staff as well as individual departments. We train the medical staff at over 600 hospitals, surgi-centers, medical offices, dental offices, walk-in medial offices, anesthesia groups, major drug stores, and military bases throughout Long Island, New York City, and Westchester. We also train and certify medical students, PA students, NP students, and students in the allied health professions, at several colleges and universities. Many continue to come from different parts of the country to take our classes.

Our Publishing Adventure Begins

As our students moved around the country, our study guides went with them. This national exposure created a demand for our study guides throughout the fifty states and the entire English speaking world. This demand was just the push we needed to start our own publishing company. As college nursing professors, students, and hospital education departments from around the country began calling us requesting to purchase our study guides, we began printing them at home and sending them out as fast as physically possible.

But the demand became too great and too time consuming. So we then hired a professional printing company to print them for us in large quantities. Luckily, the internet came along, and then the new-media publishing revolution began. So we jumped in with both feet and with our eyes and ears wide open.

Dedication

• We dedicate this book to healthcare professionals everywhere who have dedicated their life to helping those in need; and,

• To healthcare students who do not yet realize the potential and importance of the career they have chosen; and,

• To our students all over Long Island and New York City (and those that have spread out over the 50 states), and our readers, including the American military medical personnel, all over the world, that work every day at making their career a success and our world a much better place in which to live;

• To Christine Molinari, RN, who works with us everday, contacting and registering our students, along with organizing and teaching the classes too; and,

• Finally, we dedicate this book to you all with our love, appreciation, and thanks for allowing us to be a part of your lives.

Legal Disclaimer

This book is presented solely for educational purposes for healthcare professionals and healthcare students. This book is not meant to be used by non-healthcare persons, nor should it be used to diagnose or treat any medical condition. For diagnosis or treatment of any medical problem, consult your own physician. The publisher and authors are not responsible for any specific health needs that may require medical supervision and are not liable for any damages or negative consequences from any treatment, action, application, or preparation, to any person reading or following the information in this book. Neither the American Heart Association (AHA), nor the American Red Cross (ARC), endorse this publication.

References are provided for informational purposes only and do not constitute endorsement of any websites or other sources. Readers should be aware that the websites and links listed in this book may change at any time, and without notice.

Bibliography

Sinz, Elizabeth, ed. (2016). *Basic Life Support (BLS) Providers: Manual.* American Heart Association.

Kunz, Michele G. (2013). *Zombie Notes Study Charts: BLS Vocabulary.* Dickson Keanaghan, LLC.

Kunz, Michele G. (2016). *Zombie Notes Study Charts: BLS Certification Exam Prep.* Dickson Keanaghan, LLC.

Acknowledgements

In preparing to write this acknowledgments section, a flood of memories came back to me of the many people that were part of my development as a nurse and nursing educator. I have been developing my skills as a nurse, and nurse educator, for over 32 years. And I still continue to develop my skills every day. I would like to tell you about some of the people that played an important part of my professional development.

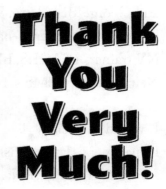

My first CPR and first-aide course was at The College of Staten Island, in New York City, (then it was called Staten Island Community College), taught by Ira Sweet, in 1976. To this day I use his teaching techniques to motivate my students to be successful healthcare professionals. He inspired me, and everyone in the class, by including real-life on-the-job stories into his lecture.

When I became an ICU nurse at Staten Island Hospital, in New York City, in 1980, I had the opportunity to work with and learn from many highly skilled critical care nurses. The one that stood out the most was my nursing preceptor Laura Gasparis-Von Frolio. She was a very dynamic patient-advocate and a brilliant nurse. After taking a four-day AHA-BLS Instructor Course at Beth Israel Medical Center, in New York City, in 1984, Gasparis and I began to teach classes to dental and medical offices and to the community. We called our little training company CPR Associates.

I loved teaching these classes and wanted to teach many more. Luckily, in 1984, my SIH-ICU co-worker and friend Rosemary Egitto-Burda read about an open position for CPR Coordinator at Long Island College Hospital, in Brooklyn. I interviewed for this position and was accepted. I was to remain at LICH as an educator for the next 25 years (my first 13 years as a Staff-Development Instructor and CPR Coordinator; my last 12 years as Director of Nursing Education and Informatics).

During my time at LICH, 1984-2009, I was also involved in American Heart Association (AHA) program developments as a Committee Member at The Regional Emergency

Medical Services Council, of NY (REMSCO). It was the only Community Training Center (CTC) in NYC at the time (1980's). Names that stand out from those days are Nancy and George Benedetto, Virginia Klunder, Mary Gallagher, and Ed Stapleton. Our group looked at the evidence-based practice and science to develop the best training programs for NY trainers in ACLS, BLS, and PALS. This organization also provided guidelines for the New York City EMS services.

I would especially like thank to my LICH co-workers in the Nursing Education Department: Esme Elisson, RN-NP, Emergency Department Clinical Nurse Specialist; Lorraine Woltman, RN; and, and Louisa Travers, RN. I worked closely with these amazingly talented nursing educators teaching the nurses and other healthcare professionals for 25 years. Many of these years included the late Lynn Hahn, RN. Lynn was a very experienced and professional nurse whose skills I always admired.

I am especially proud of Robin Ndiaye, the administrative secretary for the Nursing Department. She also took the BLS Instructor Course and has been teaching CPR to the staff and community for many years. These woman would flex their hours and work with manikins on the floor for hours and hours in order to get our staff certified. We would then clean the manikins for another two hours – and we always had a good time doing it together.

I would also like to thank my good friend and fellow nurse Christine Molinari. We started together in critical care on Staten Island. And, coincidentally, both of our families moved out to Long Island to work and live. We teach many, many classes together. She always brings great humor, and a great work ethic, to all of my classes. Christine has always made my students feel comfortable and relaxed with a friendly learning environment.

More than anyone else, I must thank my best friend and husband, Joseph. When Joe and I met in 1984, I was working full-time in the Intensive Care Unit at Staten Island Hospital, in New York City, and teaching a few classes in Brooklyn and Queens, on the side. Joe was building his first start-up company on Long Island, and assisting me with the classes. Around 1988 the two of us took a part-time job at B and G, a nursing service in Brooklyn, where we taught certification classes to nurses and physicians. I taught the classes, and Joe learned about managing the business, the classes, the students, the classroom, the other instructors, and the equipment.

Eventually we started to teach more classes on our own. We very quickly built a dedicated following of nurses and physicians throughout New York City and Long Island. We then started to grow the company very quickly by training and certifying the medical staff at several medical offices - and then entire hospitals. Amazingly, we now train and certify medical professionals and students in over 600 hospitals, medical offices, surgi-centers, universities, and military bases, throughout Long Island, New York City, and Westchester.

Our business would not be as successful as it is without the both of us working together. Right from the beginning Joe brought all his business experience and entrepreneurial fortitude into our operation. Joe had been developing his business skills and work-ethic from a very young age. He has worked very hard at making our business professional, successful, and strong. Over these last 32 years, I have perfected the teaching part of our operation, and he has perfected the marketing, management, and financial side.

He is also the one that makes it possible for our little training business to reach out and connect with many thousands of healthcare professionals every day of the year, all over the world. He has an amazing ability to put all the information I throw at him into a practical and beautiful format. He is able to make our publications, websites, and videos, in such a way that our students are able learn the material with ease. And most recently a Facebook page called "The Nurse Eductor Michele Kunz" where I connect and share with my students every day.

Joe has been our business manager since 1984. In 2003, we expanded our business once again, and named it Dickson Keanaghan, which are names from Joe's family. Joe became the President and CEO of our new corporation, and he officially became Director of Operations for our training company. In these roles he is responsible for all finance, marketing, and business development. Our business has been a wonderful 32 year learning experience and journey.

Michele G. Kunz
Long Island, New York

Praise For The *Zombie Notes Study Charts* And For Michele And Her Classes

"Michele's YouTube videos were terrific! Clear, concise, and very helpful. The *Zombie Notes* are the best way to study and review this information - and actually learn it. The groupings and mnemonics make it easy to apply in real patient situations. In Michele's class I actually learned pertinent facts that translate into real practice. It really doesn't get any better than Michele's class - quick, convenient, and very meaningful."
Denise May, RN, Winthrop University Hospital, Mineola, NY

"I took Michele's class with all of my co-workers here at our office. I loved the *Zombie Notes Study Charts*. They were very helpful. Michele has a great personality and is perfect for teaching nurses. I really enjoyed her class and I look forward to taking her other classes."
Erin Cunningham, RN, Long Island Lung Center, Bay Shore, NY

"The YouTube videos were great. I have been to Michele's classes in the past. The *Zombie Notes Study Charts* were short, concise, and to the point, but full of pertinent information. I like that Michele provided us with the Zombie Notes. Michele is full of practical and useful information and very funny."
Kate Burke, RN, Cohen Children's Medical Center of New York, New York City, NY

"Michele's videos were the first time I was seeing ECG strips. Because of her videos, I showed up to her class well prepared. They helped make the class much easier to understand. I rewrote the *Zombie Notes* twice to help memorize them. By going back and re-reading what I wrote, while watching the videos, was helping me to understand them. I am applying for my clinical ladder and Michele's class was a requirement. I am glad I learned this material. Michele kept the class fun and interesting. The notes and slides were broken down into very easy to understand segments."
Christine Chambers, Good Samaritan Hospital, West Islip, NY

"Michele's program has an excellent presentation and an enjoyable format. Her program is interactive and an excellent discussion that can't be offered by a computer-based program."
Dr. Paul Epstein, NAPA, North Shore - Long Island Jewish Medical Center, Manhasset, NY

"I have already been to Michele's classes three times. The *Zombie Notes* are the best memorization guide available. Michele is also the best educator around, by far. We ask her to teach our office every time."
Dr. Steven Macharola, Island Eye Surgi-Center, Carle Place, NY

"I watched Michele's videos. They helped me know what to expect and how to prepare for class. I have been to Michele's classes in the past. I loved the *Zombie Notes*. Everyone I know uses them to study for the PA boards. I liked the pace of Michele's class, and the hands-on-experience we gained."
Samanta Prinzing, PA, Montefiore Hospital, Manhattan, NY

"Michele's videos were awesome. My friends at Brookhaven Hospital told me about Michele's classes. The *Zombie Notes* were also awesome. They really helped me retain the information. The class was excellent and I learned a lot. The class is very concise and informative. Michele is a great instructor. Thank you Michele."
Ken Daniels, RN, Jamaica Hospital, Queens, NY

"I learned about Michele's classes from a co-worker. The videos were very helpful in understanding the material. Michele made the class a lot of fun, but we also gained a lot of knowledge. Michele had an excellent knowledge of the material and was able to help me understand the info."
Sandra Fernandez, RN, Long Island Center for Digestive Health, Garden City, NY

"I learned about Michele's classes from a co-worker. Her *Zombie Notes* were great - brief and to the point. Michele was very easy to understand. I felt much more confident in the subject matter by the time I finished her class. I loved Michele's class so much. I felt more relaxed than when I first took ACLS with a different instructor."
Doreen Cooney, RN, Nassau University Medical Center, East Meadow, NY

"I have taken Michele's classes in the past and returned to take her ACLS class again. Her class was informative, timely, and very pertinent."
Barbara Kusky, RN, Bay Pines VA Hospital, Bay Pines, FL

"Michele's class is concise, to the point, very informative, and very entertaining."
Laurie Savoia, RN, Long Island Center for Digestive Health, Garden City, NY

"I come to Michele Kunz every time I need an AHA class because she is the greatest instructor, educator, teacher, nursing brain to ever walk on the planet."
Andrea LaFata, RN, Nursing Supervisor, Good Samaritan Hospital, West Islip, NY

"I liked Michele's YouTube videos very much. They were very informative. After watching, everything began to "click", and I began to understand much more. Michele was very informative, and student friendly. She is very geared to teaching and helping, not failing people."
Laura Monas, RN, Cohen's Children's Medical Center Of New York, at Long Island Jewish Medical Center, Lake Success, NY

"Michele's YouTube videos made it very easy for me to prepare for the class. The *Zombie Notes Study Charts* were excellent, and highlighted all the important information. Michele is very personable, and made learning the material less stressful."
Madaline Safrey, RN, St. Joseph's Hospital, Bethpage, NY

"I liked Michele's YouTube videos. The *Zombie Notes Study Charts* were very helpful. Her class is very interactive and very friendly. Everything was excellent."
Dr. Araz Ibragimov, Kings County Hospital, Brooklyn, NY

"The *Zombie Notes Study Charts* were an excellent study guide. It goes straight to the important stuff."
Dr. Yimar Berrios, Kings County Hospital, Brooklyn, NY

"Thank you very much Michele! I always look forward to your classes. You truly have a gift. Making people laugh and enjoy learning at the same time is a beautiful thing."
Rosemary Fine, RN, North Shore-Long Island Jewish Medical Center, Lake Success, NY

"My nursing professor Cathy Jansen at Nassau Community College recommended that I take Michele's class for ACLS. Professor Jansen has previously taken Michele's ACLS class. I really enjoyed Michele's YouTube videos tremendously. And her *Zombie Notes Study Charts* were also a great way to comprehend the study material beforehand. As a student nurse, I have a great interest in critical care, which is Michele's specialty. Michele is phenomenal. Her class was broken up between the lecture, the video, the written test, and the hands-on exam."
Jessica Joseph, Nursing student at Nassau Community College, Garden City, NY

"Michele's YouTube videos were terrific! Clear, concise, and very helpful. The *Zombie Notes Study Charts* are the best way to study and review this information – and actually learn it. The groupings and mnemonics make it easy to apply in real patient situations. In Michele's class I actually learned pertinent facts that translate into real practice. It really doesn't get any better than Michele's class – quick, convenient, and meaningful."
Denise May, Winthrop University Hospital, Mineola, NY

Request For Testimonials

We are looking for short testimonials about this book to be used in all of our promotional material, on our websites, and possibly here in this book.

It should be a three to five sentence long statement about this book and how it has helped you with passing the certification exam. Please be as specific and as detailed as possible. You can see examples of great testimonials inside the book.

Please include your name, title, hospital or company name, and town and state. You are also welcome to include a small picture of yourself, as well as a link to your website.

You can quickly and easily send us your testimonial by email at: MKunz@TheNurseEducator.com.

By sending us your testimonial, you are giving us permission to use it in any and all of our advertising and marketing programs.

Thank you very much. We greatly appreciate your help with this.

Joe & Michele Kunz

"I just completed Michele's ACLS and BLS certification classes. I loved the *Zombie Notes Study Charts*. They streamlined the key facts needed to provide effective ACLS and BLS to my patients – and were a big help when preparing for the class and exam. I also enjoyed Michele's YouTube videos. I was very impressed with how easy Michele's videos made it for me to understand the topics we needed to know about for the class. Michele's class was very relaxed, yet very professional."
Linda Stio, RN, Neurological Surgery, PC, Long Island, NY

Colophon

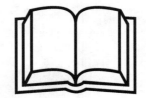

- Interior text originally created in MS Word
- Final book created in Adobe InDesign CC
- All fonts from Adobe Typekit

- All text and bullets set in Adobe Caslon Pro
- Page headers set in Myriad Pro
- Graphics and cover created in Adobe Illustrator CC

- Cover colors created in Adobe Color CC
- Cover fonts are Trajan Pro 3, and Myriad Pro
- Photographs created in Adobe Photoshop CC

- Finished book and cover converted to PDF using Adobe Acrobat Pro DC
- CIP data block created by librarian and publisher Adrienne Bashista, cipblock.com
- Trademarks filed and managed by attorney Kelly Talcott, kdtalcott.com

- Paperback book printed and bound by Lightning Source
- Paperback book distibution by Lightning Source, and Ingram
- Online retail sales by Amazon

Notes

Book Publishing Codes and Subject Headings for this Publication

BISAC EDI-Codes and Subject Headings:
• MED026000 MEDICAL / Emergency Medicine
• MED024000 MEDICAL / Education & Training
• MED086000 MEDICAL / Test Preparation & Review

Thema Codes and Subject Headings:
• Medicine & Nursing
• MQF: First Aid & Paramedical Services
• MR: Medical study & revision guides & reference material
• 4CP: For vocational / professional education

Amazon Best Sellers Rank Subject Headings:
• Books > Textbooks > Medicine & Health Sciences > Medicine > Clinical > Cardiology
• Books > Textbooks > Medicine & Health Sciences > Medicine > Clinical > Emergency Medicine
• Books > Medical Books > Medicine > Internal Medicine > Emergency
• Books > Medical Books > Medicine > Internal Medicine > Pathology > Diseases > Cardiovascular
• Books > Textbooks > Medicine & Health Sciences > Nursing > Test Preparation & Review
• Books > Cardiovascular
• Books > BLS
• Books > CPR

Bookstore Shelving / Sales Category:
• Medical > Test Preparation & Review

This Book is Available From:
• Amazon
• Ingram

Dickson Keanaghan
Medical Publications

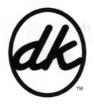

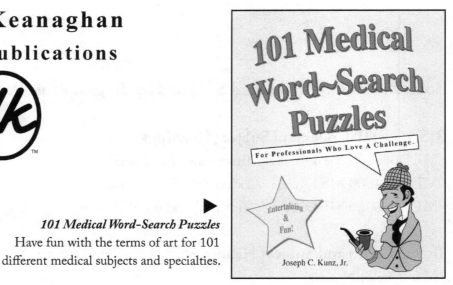

▶

101 Medical Word-Search Puzzles
Have fun with the terms of art for 101
different medical subjects and specialties.

▶

Notes on Nursing: What It Is & What It Is Not
The student edition of the best selling and most
important nursing book ever written, by the
"Mother of Modern Nursing" Florence Nightingale.

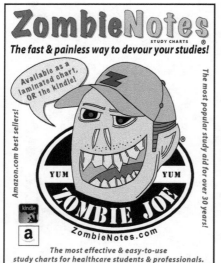

◀

The Zombie Notes Study Charts
ALL are current for 2017.
Each one is two pages long, and packed with info.
They can be downloaded for the kindle,
or purchased as a laminated card-stock.
Subjects: ACLS, BLS, PALS, NRP, ECG, Shock,
Bradycardia, ABG, and more related to these subjects.

Dickson Keanaghan
Medical Publications

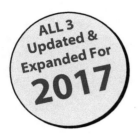

ALL 3
Updated &
Expanded For
2017

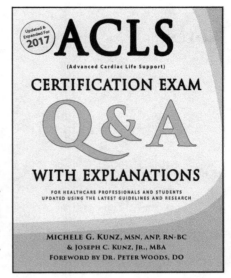

▶

ACLS Certification Exam Q&A With Explanations
Publication Date: November 2016
101 practice questions that cover every possible medical and nursing scenario and topic on the ACLS certification exam.

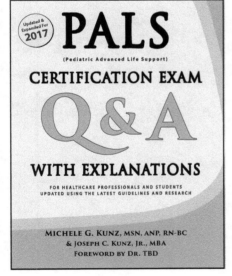

◀

PALS Certification Exam Q&A With Explanations
Publication Date: Mid-2017
101 practice questions that cover every possible medical and nursing scenario and topic on the PALS certification exam.

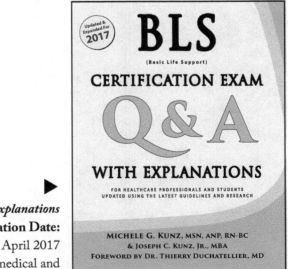

▶

BLS Certification Exam Q&A With Explanations
Publication Date:
April 2017
101 practice questions that cover every possible medical and nursing scenario and topic on the BLS certification exam.

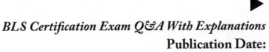

Notes

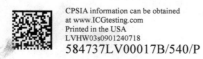

9 781933 230801